MW00490494

Healing Autoimmune Disease

A plan to help your immune system and reduce inflammation

By

Sandra Cabot MD
and
Margaret Jasinska ND

www.sandracabot.com

www.liverdoctor.com

Published in the United States by SCB International Inc.
 PO Box 5070, Glendale Phoenix, AZ 85312-5070
Telephone 623 334 3232

Distributed in the UK & Europe by
Roundhouse Group, Maritime House,
Basin Road North, Hove BN41 1WR
T. 01273 704 962 F. 01273 704 963
W. www.roundhousegroup.co.uk
E. alan@roundhousegroup.co.uk

www.sandracabot.com   www.liverdoctor.com
ISBN 978-1-936609-39-0

HEA039090   HEALTH & FITNESS / Diseases / Immune & Autoimmune
HEA006000   HEALTH & FITNESS / Diet & Nutrition / Diets

Typesetting and cover design by Victoria Herrera.

Contents

About the Authors..7

Introduction...8

Chapter One..13

    What is autoimmune disease?...13

Chapter Two...16

    Types of autoimmune diseases...16

    List of autoimmune diseases...18

Chapter Three..28

    What causes autoimmune disease?...28

    Genetics...29

    Infections...32

    Heavy metals...40

    Silicone..43

    Vaccinations..49

    Drugs/medication..55

    Stress...55

    Postpartum thyroiditis..62

    Nutritional deficiencies...65

    Food sensitivities..70

Chapter Four..73

    The role of the gut and liver in autoimmune disease....................................73

    Leaky gut syndrome..73

    What causes a leaky gut?..80

    How to fix a leaky gut...82

    Dysbiosis and small intestinal bacterial overgrowth (SIBO).......................84

    What functions does your gut microbiome perform for you?.......................85

Symptoms of Small Intestinal Bacterial Overgrowth (SIBO)........................ 90

Causes of Small Intestinal Bacterial Overgrowth (SIBO) 91

How to overcome SIBO 97

You may have a yeast or fungal overgrowth 100

Fix your digestion...104

The importance of stomach acid 105

The importance of bile 110

The importance of digestive enzymes 112

The impact of autoimmune disease on liver health...113

Chapter Five...**116**

Problematic foods for anyone with autoimmune disease...............................116

The problem with gluten and other grains...117

Harmful effects of lectins..121

The problem with legumes...125

The problem with dairy products 126

Nightshade vegetables...129

The problem with eggs...130

Nuts and seeds 132

Harmful effects of sugar on the immune system..133

Chapter Six **134**

Foods to eat to heal autoimmune disease 134

Vegetables...135

Fruit 138

Animal protein..141

Healthy fats 145

Nuts and seeds 149

Superfoods and recipes for healing autoimmune disease..............................149

Fermented vegetables..149

Offal, cartilage and marrow 153

Bone Broth 158

Coconut oil 160

Stage 1 Autoimmune Eating Plan 164

Stage 2 Autoimmune Eating Plan 167

Low FODMAP diet 168

Additional sources of recipes 170

Chapter Seven **172**

Supportive supplements for overcoming autoimmune disease 172

Vitamin D 173

St Mary's thistle/Silybum marianum (Milk thistle) 176

Turmeric (Curcuma longa) 177

Selenium 178

N-acetyl cysteine 180

Zinc 181

Glutamine 182

MSM (Methyl Sulphonyl Methane) 183

Bupleurum falcatum 184

Berberine 184

Magnesium 185

Probiotics 186

Omega 3 essential fatty acids 187

Vitamin A 188

Vitamin C 189

Low dose naltrexone 190

Chapter Eight **192**

Troubleshooting: 192

What to do when the recommendations aren't working 192

You may have a parasitic gut infection 192

Histamine intolerance 195

What to do if cravings get out of control 198

How to overcome adrenal gland exhaustion 201

How to handle an autoimmune flare 203

Chapter Nine **206**

Tests required in the diagnosis and monitoring of

autoimmune disease 206

Chapter Ten...**214**

Case studies of patients who have reversed their

autoimmune disease 214

Chapter Eleven...**228**

The Conventional medical treatment of autoimmune disease.................228

Glossary 235

References 238

Index 245

About the Authors

Sandra Cabot MD

Dr Sandra Cabot is the author of thirty books on health, including the famous Liver Cleansing Diet book which has sold over 2 million copies and is translated into 6 languages. She graduated with Honours in Medicine and Surgery in 1975 from Adelaide University, South Australia. During the 1980s Sandra spent considerable time working in the Department of Obstetrics and Gynaecology in a large missionary hospital in the Himalayan foothills of India.

Dr Cabot has lectured for the American Liver Foundation, The Primary Biliary Cirrhosis Society and The Hepatitis C Council of Australia where she was the protagonist in the great debate "Does the liver need a good cleanse?"

Dr Cabot regularly conducts health seminars and is involved in raising funds for various charities all over Australia. She is an Angel Flight pilot who donates her time and aircraft to transport disadvantaged patients.

Margaret Jasinska ND

Margaret Jasinska is a naturopath with more than eighteen years of clinical experience. Margaret has co-authored eight books with Dr Cabot. She divides her time between seeing patients at Dr Cabot's clinic, writing and researching new developments in health and medicine.

Margaret's main area of interest is in digestive and immune system disorders. She greatly enjoys empowering individuals to improve their health by giving them the tools and knowledge to lead healthier lives. Health and wellness is a great passion and hobby of hers.

Being diagnosed with celiac disease is what inspired Margaret to become a naturopath.

Introduction

Autoimmune disease is becoming an increasingly significant problem in the United States and around the world. Autoimmune diseases are a broad range of conditions where a person's immune system launches an attack against their own cells, tissues and/or organs. This results in inflammation throughout the body, and significant damage to specific parts of the body.

There are officially 81 different autoimmune diseases, with around another 20 or so diseases considered to have an autoimmune component. Increasingly, diseases that were once considered idiopathic (of unknown origin), are now being labelled autoimmune.

Autoimmune diseases range from very common to extremely rare diseases. Some autoimmune diseases affect mainly one part of the body (such as autoimmune thyroid disease, multiple sclerosis and type 1 diabetes); others affect many parts of the body (such as systemic lupus erythematosus, rheumatoid arthritis and scleroderma).

The incidence of autoimmune disease is exploding at a frightening pace

It affects approximately 1 in 20 people and is one of the most significant health issues in Australia and New Zealand[1]. Approximately 50 million people in the United States suffer with an autoimmune disease.

What has happened to cause this explosion? Why does a person's immune system turn on themselves and start attacking healthy organs and tissues? The answer is complicated and multifactorial, but researchers are uncovering clues at a rapid pace. The information we've shared with you in this book is based on the latest research into the function of the immune system and also our clinical experience with helping patients with autoimmune disease.

Our aim in writing this book is to teach you and empower you. You have an enormous amount of control over the quality of your health and the severity of your autoimmune disease. We want to give you as much information as possible because we believe if you have the most up-to-date knowledge, you're more likely to make wise and informed decisions that benefit your health and, ultimately, your life.

Your doctor may have told you nothing can be done to heal autoimmune disease and that you'll just have to manage your symptoms with a cocktail of medications for the rest of your life. You may have been told autoimmune disease is genetic and there's nothing you can do about it because you've got faulty genes and you'll just have to learn to live with them. Yes, genes do play an important role in autoimmune disease but they are only one piece of the puzzle, and a small one at that.

Research shows that 70 to 95 percent of the risk of developing autoimmune disease comes from your environment, not your genes.

Environment refers to foods you eat, chemicals you're exposed to or stress you're subjected to. The good news is you have a great deal of control over your environment, regardless of the genes you've inherited.

In the past, most people thought there was nothing that could be done to overcome an autoimmune disease. Once you've got it, you'll have it for life and it will probably get worse. We now know that's not the truth. It is possible to experience a significant improvement in your health.

At the very least, you should be able to reduce your symptoms, reduce pain and improve your energy level. At best, you may be able to halt the autoimmune disease, stop autoantibody production and enable the repair of damaged organs or tissues in your body.

There is quite a bit of controversy over whether or not autoimmune disease can be cured, or if the patient just stays in remission. It really doesn't matter what terminology we use; we want you to know that it is possible to significantly improve your health and improve your quality of life.

We have included a chapter with real life case studies from our clinic. These are the stories of people who have reversed their autoimmune disease. You may be able to relate to them, and we truly hope you find them inspiring. Reading their stories will show you what is possible.

If you haven't heard of Dr Terry Wahls, we strongly suggest you look her up on the internet. She is an American doctor who reversed a severe form of progressive multiple sclerosis. She has done a TEDx talk called **'Minding your mitochondria'** which has received more than 2 million views on the internet. Dr Wahls went from a wheelchair to riding her bike and working full time. Viewing the images in her video presentation is very inspirational. She used the same dietary principles to reverse multiple sclerosis as we use in our clinics and have detailed for you in this book.

The guidelines in our book will help you regardless of which autoimmune disease you have, because the underlying immune dysfunction is the same for each disease, therefore the basic treatment is the same. The conventional medical treatment of autoimmune disease leaves a lot to be desired and many people choose to discontinue treatment because the side effects are worse than the disease.

Conventional treatment focuses on drugs that create immunosuppression. Suppressing the immune system can be very effective for reducing the symptoms of autoimmune disease, and protecting organs from damage, but in the long term, can have harmful side effects such as an increased risk of infections or cancer.

Many people are diagnosed with a disease but not told it is autoimmune. For example, a person with an underactive thyroid gland is prescribed thyroid hormone, but no mention is given to the actual cause of the disease, which is autoimmune destruction of the thyroid gland. This is a shame because it means the patient doesn't really understand the nature of their disease and what they could be doing about it. Also, if we don't address the underlying immune dysfunction, a person is much more prone to developing a second or third autoimmune disease.

Additionally, new research is uncovering an autoimmune component in diseases where the cause was always considered a mystery

For example, a study was published in 2012 in the medical journal Autoimmunity Reviews titled "Is there an association between autoimmunity and endometriosis?" After a thorough review of the literature, the authors concluded that endometriosis fulfills most of the classification criteria for autoimmune disease, including blood markers of inflammatory cytokines and tissue specific autoantibodies. They also noted that endometriosis often occurs with other autoimmune conditions such as autoimmune thyroid disease and inflammatory bowel disease.

There is new and exciting research linking some forms of schizophrenia and Parkinson's disease to autoimmunity. It will be very interesting to follow research in this field in the coming years.

Most surprising of all, a paper appeared in the journal Bio Med Central Medicine called "Is atherosclerosis an autoimmune disease?". People don't get clogged arteries from eating too much fat; atherosclerosis is far more complex than that. It is not merely a plumbing problem. It has recently been uncovered that some people produce antibodies against LDL cholesterol particles, and these antibodies can cause autoimmune destruction to the inner lining of arteries. Autoimmunity definitely plays a major role in the development of coronary artery disease because it has been known for a long time that people with rheumatoid arthritis and lupus suffer from heart attacks much more frequently; even if they're slim and fit. In fact, people with lupus are 50 times more likely to have a heart attack than people of the same age who don't have lupus.

As mentioned, autoimmune disease is incredibly common. Most people don't die specifically from it though; it just significantly reduces their quality of life.

Having an autoimmune disease usually causes symptoms like fatigue, unrefreshing sleep, pain, brain fog and low mood.

It's very difficult to put up with these symptoms long term, while dealing with a busy life and the inescapable stress that usually goes with it.

It is our sincerest wish that reading this book will offer you the knowledge and tools you need to improve your health and your life. Good health really is your greatest asset; it's so important for leading a productive and enjoyable life. Hopefully you'll find the answers you're looking for in this book.

If you have any questions after reading this book, we'd love you to get in touch with us. We have a range of personalised services that may help you. You can call our Health Advisory line and speak to a naturopath on 623 334 3232. Our email address is contact@liverdoctor.com

Chapter One

What is autoimmune disease?

Autoimmune disease means that your body's immune cells become confused and start attacking your own body. Auto means self. Virtually any organ or tissue in the body can be attacked. If you have an autoimmune disease, your immune system literally believes that a component of your own body is a harmful foreign invader that shouldn't be there and needs to be destroyed. Therefore your immune cells produce what is known as autoantibodies.

Rheumatoid arthritis, Hashimoto's thyroiditis (causing an underactive thyroid gland), psoriasis, lupus and ulcerative colitis are examples of common autoimmune diseases.

In all autoimmune conditions, there is an imbalance in the immune system

Pro-inflammatory white blood cells are overactive, whereas inflammation-suppressing cells and regulatory immune cells are underactive. The result is an unabated attack on your own organs and tissues.

It's not just antibodies that your immune cells produce if you suffer with autoimmune disease; a whole host of inflammatory chemicals are also made, particularly inflammatory cytokines. Cytokines are signalling molecules that allow white blood cells to communicate with each other about the nature and location of a foreign invasion or injury. In the case of autoimmune disease, your healthy organs are mistaken as an invader.

The excessive immune activity in the body of someone affected by autoimmune disease means there is far too much inflammation in the body. Autoimmune disease can produce a great deal of pain and tissue dysfunction, but the symptoms vary greatly depending on which specific part of the body is affected. The inflammation generated usually produces a lot of fatigue. The inflammatory chemicals also end up causing collateral damage to other parts of the body that were never targeted in the initial assault. The inflammation generates free radical damage and oxidative stress, which basically causes wear and tear to your body.

This means autoimmune disease can speed up the rate of ageing and raise the risk of a number of diseases triggered by inflammation such as heart disease and cancer.

How common is autoimmune disease?

Autoimmune disease is becoming increasingly common. In Australia and New Zealand it affects approximately one in 20 people. According to the American Autoimmune Related Diseases Association, there are approximately 50 million people in the United States with autoimmune disease. After cardiovascular disease and cancer, autoimmune diseases are the most common class of illness in the United States[2].

Autoimmune disease can occur in anybody. Some diseases, such as type 1 diabetes are most common in children, whereas rheumatoid arthritis is more common in older people. Most autoimmune diseases are far more common in women than men; in fact, 78.8 percent of all cases of autoimmune disease occur in women[3]. It's thought this is because of the effects female hormones have on the immune system. Autoimmune diseases fall into the top 10 causes of death for women in all age groups up to 64 years[4]. Fortunately, most people don't die from their autoimmune disease. It just makes life unpleasant because of the fatigue, pain, unrefreshing sleep and other common symptoms.

The individuals most at risk of developing an autoimmune disease are women between the ages of 20 and 40. There are a few autoimmune diseases more common in men, and these include type 1 diabetes,

Graves' disease, ankylosing spondylitis and autoimmune myocarditis.

Unfortunately, once you have developed an autoimmune disease, you are far more likely to develop a second, third or even more autoimmune diseases. The majority of the patients who come to our clinic have more than one autoimmune disease. It is vital to address the underlying imbalance in the immune system, otherwise the condition will just continue to express itself in new ways.

The other problem is there are a large number of people with undiagnosed autoimmune disease. They are going about their life, feeling unwell, feeling chronically tired but don't know why. Their doctor has ordered a few basic blood tests, which haven't picked up the disease, so the patient continues to suffer. In many cases, there is quite a long lag time between first feeling unwell and being officially diagnosed with an autoimmune disease. This is quite typical in the case of systemic lupus erythematosus.

In the next chapter we have listed the most common symptoms of the earliest stages of autoimmunity; before a specific disease is diagnosed. You may recognise some of these symptoms and realise you've felt this way for a long time.

Chapter Two

Types of autoimmune diseases

According to the National Institutes of Health, there are at least 81 confirmed autoimmune diseases. However, there are approximately 100 diseases that are suspected to be autoimmune, or have an autoimmune component but for which definitive evidence is not yet available.

Professor Yehuda Shoenfeld is a world leader in the research on autoimmune disease. He is a clinician at the Zabludowitz Center of Autoimmune Diseases, Sheba-Medical Center, Tel Aviv University, Israel. He has published more than 1600 scientific papers and has authored 25 books on the subject of autoimmune disease. He is also the editor of the Journal of Autoimmunity.

Professor Shoenfeld is well known for saying: "Everything is autoimmune unless proven otherwise". There is a lot of wisdom in that statement when you consider that recent studies have uncovered an autoimmune component in schizophrenia, Parkinson's disease, epilepsy and atherosclerosis.

Additionally, diseases that were once called idiopathic (a medical term that means of unknown origin) are increasingly discovered to be autoimmune

For example, the medical name for abnormally low platelet levels in the bloodstream is ITP (Idiopathic Thrombocytopenia). This disease is now known to be autoimmune and the name has been changed to autoimmune thrombocytopenic purpura. Type 1 diabetes was once called idiopathic, whereas now it is known to be autoimmune.

What are the most common autoimmune diseases?

The most common autoimmune diseases are Hashimoto's thyroiditis (causes an underactive thyroid gland) and psoriasis (causes a skin rash). The interesting table below highlights the prevalence of the other most common autoimmune diseases.

Disease	Body part affected	Prevalence in Population per 100,000
Hashimoto's thyroiditis	Thyroid gland	9,460
Psoriasis	Skin	2,020
Graves' disease	Thyroid gland	1,120
Rheumatoid arthritis	Joints	920
Uveitis	Eye	850
Vitiligo	Skin	740
Lupus erythematosus	Connective tissue	510
Celiac disease	Small intestine	400
Autoimmune urticaria (hives)	Skin	330
Crohn's disease	Gastrointestinal tract	184
Alopecia areata	Hair follicles	170
Multiple sclerosis	Brain, nerves	140
Ankylosing spondylitis	Spine and sacroiliac joints	129
Type 1 diabetes	Pancreas	120
Scleroderma	Skin and connective tissue	110
Ulcerative colitis	Colon	35-100

Reference: Professor Loren Cordain, 2010.

List of autoimmune diseases

The following diseases are either confirmed to be autoimmune, or there is strong scientific evidence for an autoimmune component:

A

Acute brachial neuropathy (also known as Parsonage-Turner syndrome)

Acute disseminated encephalomyelitis

Acute necrotising haemorrhagic leukoencephalitis

Addison's disease

Allergic granulomatosis

Alopecia areata

Amyloidosis (some forms)

Ankylosing spondylitis

Antiphospholipid syndrome

Aplastic anaemia

Atrophic polychondritis

Autoimmune angioedema

Autoimmune haemolytic anaemia

Autoimmune hepatitis

Autoimmune inner ear disease (AIED)

Autoimmune orchitis

Autoimmune pancreatitis

Autoimmune peripheral neuropathy

Autoimmune polyendocrine syndrome (APS)

Autoimmune polyendocrine syndrome (Type 1, 2 or 3)

Autoimmune progesterone dermatitis

B

Balo concentric sclerosis (very similar to multiple sclerosis)

Behcet's disease

Bickerstaff's encephalitis

Brachial plexus neuropathy (Parsonage-Turner syndrome)

Bullous pemphigoid

C

Castleman's disease

Cerebral amyloid angiopathy

Chilblains

Chronic inflammatory demyelinating polyneuropathy

Chronic recurrent multifocal osteomyelitis

Churg-Strauss syndrome (allergic granulomatosis)

Cicatricial pemphigoid

Celiac disease

Cogan's syndrome

Cold agglutinin disease (a type of haemolytic anaemia)

Complex regional pain syndrome

CREST syndrome (limited systemic sclerosis)

Crohn's disease

Cryoglobulinaemia (some forms)

D

Dermatitis herpetiformis

Dermatomyositis

Diabetes mellitus type 1

Discoid lupus erythematosus

Dressler's syndrome (post myocardial infarction syndrome)

E

Endometriosis

Eosinophilic oesophagitis

Eosinophilic fasciitis

Erythema nodosum

Erythroblastopenia

Erythromelalgia

Evans syndrome

G

Gestational pemphigoid

Giant cell arteritis (also called temporal arteritis)

Glomerulonephritis

Goodpasture's syndrome

Granuloma annulare

Granulomatosis with polyangiitis

Graves' disease

Guillain Barre syndrome

H

Hashimoto's encephalopathy

Hashimoto's thyroiditis

Henoch-Schonlein purpura

Hypogammaglobulinemia

I

Idiopathic pulmonary fibrosis

Idiopathic thrombocytopenia (ITP). Idiopathic means of unknown origin. In recent years scientists have discovered that it's caused by autoimmune disease, so that name is no longer relevant. Therefore the condition is increasingly referred to as Immune Thrombocytopenic Purpura (ITP)

IgA nephropathy

IgG4-related sclerosing disease

Inclusion body myositis

Infertiity of unknown origin is often autoimmune

Intermediate uveitis

Interstitial cystitis

K

Kawasaki syndrome

L

Lambert-Eaton myasthenic syndrome
Leukocytoclastic vasculitis
Lichen planus
Lichen sclerosus
Ligneous conjunctivitis
Linear IgA bullous dermatosis

M

Meniere's disease
Microscopic polyangiitis (microscopic polyarteritis)
Mixed connective tissue disease (MCTD)
Mooren's ulcer
Mucha-Habermann disease (also known as acute parapsoriasis)
Multiple sclerosis
Myasthenia gravis
Myositis

N

Narcolepsy
Neuromyelitis optica
Neutropenia (some forms)

O

Optic neuritis (some forms)

P

Pediatric autoimmune neuropsychiatric disorders associated with streptococcus (PANDAS)

Palindromic rheumatism

Paraneoplastic cerebellar degeneration

Paroxysmal nocturnal haemoglobinuria

Parry-Romberg syndrome (progressive hemifacial atrophy)

Pemphigus vulgaris

Perivenous encephalomyelitis

POEMS syndrome

Polyarteritis nodosa

Polymyalgia rheumatica

Polymyositis

Postpericardiotomy syndrome

Postural orthostatic tachycardia syndrome (POTS)

Primary biliary cirrhosis(PBC)

Primary sclerosing cholangitis

Psoriasis

Psoriatic arthritis

Pyoderma gangrenosum

R

Rasmussen's encephalitis (chronic focal encephalitis)

Raynaud's disease

Reactive arthritis (Reiter's syndrome)

Restless legs syndrome

Retroperitoneal fibrosis

Rheumatic fever

Rheumatoid arthritis

S

Sarcoidosis

Schnitzler syndrome

Scleritis

Scleroderma

Sjogren's syndrome

Sperm autoimmunity

Stiff person syndrome

Still's disease (juvenile rheumatoid arthritis)

Subacute bacterial endocarditis

Susac's syndrome (retinocochleocerebral vasculopathy)

Sydenham's chorea

Sympathetic ophthalmia

Systemic lupus erythematosus

T

Takayasu's arteritis

Tolosa-Hunt syndrome

Thrombocytopenic purpura

Transverse myelitis

U

Ulcerative colitis

Undifferentiated connective tissue disease

Urticaria (some types)

Urticarial vasculitis

Uveitis

V

Vitiligo

Vogt-Koyanagi-Harada syndrome

Diseases that are suspected to be autoimmune or have an autoimmune component

The following diseases seem to be partly autoimmune, or have an autoimmune component in some individuals. At the moment there is insufficient evidence to officially classify them as autoimmune. If you have one of these conditions, we recommend you follow the diet and supplement guidelines in this book.

- Fibromyalgia
- Chronic fatigue syndrome
- Schizophrenia
- Parkinson's disease
- Alzheimer's disease
- Epilepsy
- Tourette syndrome
- Autism
- Atherosclerosis and heart disease

An increasing amount of research is showing that blocked and hardened arteries that lead to heart attacks may have an autoimmune component

Studies have shown that some individuals produce anti (oxidised) LDL antibodies, which creates an immune response in the artery wall, which can then lead to fat deposition in arteries and blood clots. LDL is a type of cholesterol, traditionally known as "bad" cholesterol. Only some types of LDL cholesterol are bad though, and they are especially bad if they become oxidised.

A lack of vegetables and antioxidants in the diet, as well as consumption of oxidised omega 6 rich fats promotes the oxidation of LDL cholesterol in your body.

It is known that people with lupus have much higher rates of heart attacks, especially at a young age. In fact, people with lupus have 50 times higher rates of myocardial infarction (heart attack) than people of the same age who don't have lupus[5]. This is because production of anti-oxidised LDL cholesterol antibodies is higher in this population, and because of the inflammation itself.

All autoimmune diseases cause high levels of inflammation in the body due to the chemicals produced by immune cells. These chemicals cause wear and tear to the delicate artery walls, and this encourages fat deposition, narrowing of the arteries and propensity to form blood clots.

It is now believed that around ten percent of people that have been diagnosed with type 2 diabetes actually have an autoimmune form of the disease called "latent autoimmune diabetes in adults" (LADA).

Symptoms of autoimmune disease

Autoimmune disease is often challenging to diagnose because the symptoms can be quite vague, at least initially. Fatigue, unrefreshing sleep, foggy head, low mood as well as aches and pains are the most common symptoms. These symptoms are often put down to being stressed, overworked, not sleeping enough or just getting older. You may have visited your doctor, who performed a few basic tests that didn't reveal anything wrong, so you basically left feeling like a hypochondriac.

The symptoms of autoimmune disease can vary greatly, depending on which part of the body is affected.

The two symptoms present in virtually all autoimmune diseases are chronic fatigue and unrefreshing sleep

Some autoimmune diseases have a rapid onset with severe symptoms and therefore they are diagnosed very quickly; for example rheumatoid arthritis, autoimmune kidney disease and type 1 diabetes.

The earliest symptoms of autoimmune disease: ASIA (Autoimmune Syndrome Induced by Adjuvants)

It is now possible to determine with a fair degree of accuracy, who is likely to develop an autoimmune disease in the next few years.

Autoimmune Syndrome Induced by Adjuvants (ASIA) is a term coined by Professor Yehuda Shoenfeld of Israel. ASIA is a collection of signs and symptoms that usually predict the future development of an autoimmune disease. An adjuvant is a general term for a toxin, chemical or environmental trigger that irritates the immune system and can initiate an autoimmune disease.

Symptoms of pre-autoimmune disease may include:

- Fatigue
- Unrefreshing sleep
- Disturbed, poor quality sleep
- Cognitive impairment and/or memory loss
- Allergies
- Food intolerance
- Dry mouth
- Mild fever or feeling uncomfortably hot, particularly at night
- Muscle and/or joint aches and pains
- Muscle weakness
- Swollen glands in the neck, armpits and/or groin
- Recurrent minor infections or lingering infections
- Skin rashes
- Neurological manifestations such as numbness or tingling in the limbs
- Headaches

If you think back, you have probably experienced several of these symptoms for a long time. The earliest signs of autoimmune disease usually develop many years before a full blown autoimmune disease is diagnosed.

Research has shown that autoantibodies for specific autoimmune diseases such as lupus or Hashimoto's thyroiditis typically appear in the bloodstream for many years before a person starts to feel unwell.

Chapter Three

What causes autoimmune disease?

The short answer is several things. Firstly, you cannot develop an autoimmune disease unless you have specific genes. The tendency to develop an autoimmune disease runs in families. You won't necessarily develop the same autoimmune disease that someone in your family has; you just inherit an increased chance of developing one of them.

Just having the genes isn't enough though. You need to be exposed to one or more environmental factors that trigger off the disease. Environmental triggers include things like an infection, specific foods that your body can't tolerate, emotional stress, exposure to chemicals or toxic metals; pregnancy, a nutrient deficiency and others. The third critical component is a leaky gut (also known as increased intestinal permeability).

So you need the genes for autoimmunity, you need to have a leaky gut and then you need an environmental trigger to start off the disease process. In this chapter, we discuss the genes and environmental factors. Leaky gut is covered in great detail in Chapter Four.

A range of different environmental chemicals have been linked to the development of autoimmune disease

This is not surprising, considering our planet is becoming more polluted and the range of toxins we are exposed to on a daily basis is growing. Studies have shown that people who live near airports and people exposed to toxins in their profession (eg. printing and painting) are more likely to develop an autoimmune disease.

Genetics

A number of genes have been found to be associated with specific autoimmune diseases. Most autoimmune diseases are the result of several faulty genes; not just one gene. Very rarely in medicine is a disease the result of one specific gene mutation. Examples of those include cystic fibrosis and sickle cell anaemia. Most diseases, including autoimmune diseases are the result of several genes, which must then be activated by an environmental agent.

Even if you know you've got faulty genes because there's a strong history of autoimmune disease in your family, it is not inevitable that you'll also develop one. Research shows that 70 to 95 percent of the risk of developing autoimmune disease comes from your environment, not your genes[6]. By environment we mean your diet, your lifestyle, the chemicals you are exposed to and the emotions you experience. This is wonderful news because it means your genes are not your destiny.

You have so much power and control over what you eat and how you live your life, and this will determine whether dodgy genes you've inherited will become activated or not. Even if you already have one or more autoimmune conditions, at the very least you can reduce their severity, arrest their progression and, at best, you can reverse the disease.

Here are just a few examples of specific genes and their association with specific autoimmune diseases:

HLA DQ2 and DQ8 (celiac disease genes)

HLA stands for Human Leukocyte Antigen. Leukocytes are also known as white blood cells. Antigen refers to any substance that elicits your immune cells to produce antibodies; infectious agents like bacteria and allergens such as dust mites are common examples. HLA describes the process whereby your immune cells recognise and respond to any potential threat.

More than 90 percent of people with celiac disease have one or both of these genes. Celiac disease is an autoimmune disease triggered by the consumption of gluten. Having these genes also predisposes a person to developing other autoimmune diseases, including type 1 diabetes, dermatitis herpetiformis, Sjogren's syndrome, autoimmune hepatitis and systemic lupus erythematosus, amongst others.

It is important to note that we recommend everyone who has an autoimmune disease avoids consuming gluten, regardless of whether you have these genes or not.

Gluten has very destructive effects on the immune system and intestines of all people with autoimmune disease. Essentially it worsens leaky gut.

Therefore, if you've had a blood test for these genes and it came back negative, it simply means you don't have celiac disease. Celiac disease is just one autoimmune disease; eating gluten can still initiate or aggravate whatever other autoimmune disease you do have.

HLA-B gene mutations

A specific variant in the HLA-B gene called HLA-B27 is strongly linked with a number of different autoimmune diseases, including ankylosing spondylitis, psoriatic arthritis, inflammatory bowel disease (ulcerative colitis and Crohn's disease), iritis and acute anterior uveitis (eye diseases) and Reiter's syndrome (a type of arthritis).

This gene is found in approximately 8 percent of Caucasians, 4 percent of North Africans, 2 to 9 percent of Chinese and 0.1 to 0.5 percent of Japanese people. Interestingly, people with this gene who are infected with HIV have a significantly greater chance of survival. They are less likely to develop AIDS and die from the infection[7].

HLA-DR3 and HLA-DR15 gene mutations

These genes are most common in northern and western Europeans and they significantly increase the risk of developing autoimmune disease, particularly at a young age. The diseases most commonly associated with these genes are multiple sclerosis, myasthenia gravis, primary sclerosing cholangitis and autoimmune thyroid disease. The Epstein-Barr virus (glandular fever) is one known trigger of autoimmune disease in people with these genes.

Is it worth getting a genetic test?

In most cases, no. It is important to remember that this field of medicine is still in its infancy. We are only scratching the surface; new gene mutations are continually being discovered. According to Professor Alessio Fasano, a leading researcher into autoimmune disease, *"The more you search, the more genes come out"*. For example, in the case of systemic lupus erythematosus, so far 24 genes have been associated with the disease. A combination of genetic mutations predisposes an individual to a specific autoimmune disease.

If you are reading this book, you have probably already been diagnosed with an autoimmune disease.

Having a gene test might be interesting, and it might give you clues to which other autoimmune diseases you could develop

However, the underlying treatment of improving immune health, gut health and liver health that we've described in this book will be the same.

Having said that, there may be benefits to having a blood test for the celiac disease genes. We already recommend that everyone with an autoimmune disease avoids gluten, but having these genes means you would need to avoid gluten very strictly for life.

Any doctor can order the celiac gene test for you and it isn't expensive.

Infections

Infections are a very common trigger of autoimmune disease, and they can also cause a flare up of an existing autoimmune disease. There is a great deal of medical research to support this fact. Infection with certain bacteria, viruses, fungi or parasites doesn't cause an autoimmune disease directly, like a virus causes the flu. Instead, these infections are more like the straw that broke the camel's back. They trigger the development of an autoimmune disease in a person who was at high risk of it happening sooner or later.

Certain infections have been linked with specific autoimmune diseases

This is probably because certain viruses or bacteria closely resemble specific parts of the human body. Therefore after making antibodies against a specific bug; your immune system gets confused and starts making antibodies against your own body. This phenomenon is known as molecular mimicry and is a leading theory as to why autoimmune disease happens in the first place.

As we travel through life we are exposed to more and more infections; this, coupled with nutrient deficiencies and stress, can make autoimmune disease more likely to develop as we get older.

There are good and bad infections when it comes to autoimmune disease. Some infections are actually known to have a protective role, and it also depends on when you become infected. Infection with the stomach bacterium Helicobacter pylori in childhood can reduce the risk of autoimmune disease, while infection in adulthood may raise the risk.

The graphs on the following page illustrate how the incidence of infectious diseases is declining, while autoimmune disease is skyrocketing.

A

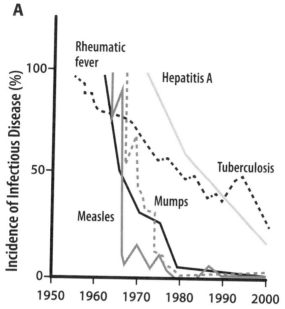

Source: Bach, *New England Journal of Medicine (2002)*

B

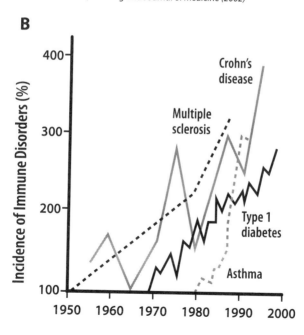

Graphs from the book "An Epidemic of Absence" by Moises Velasquez-Manoff

You have probably heard of the hygiene hypothesis. This theory states that exposure to certain bugs and microbes in childhood reduces the risk of allergies and autoimmune disease in adulthood. Children who grow up with pets or grow up on farms and are exposed to dirt usually suffer less allergies and autoimmune disease in adulthood.

Some studies have been carried out on the use of hookworms in people with inflammatory bowel disease and celiac disease with very positive results. Research participants were given capsules to swallow that contained worm eggs, and then had their inflammatory bowel disease or celiac disease monitored. Results of these studies were overwhelmingly positive; the worms dampened down excessive inflammation and balanced the immune system. In some instances, people with celiac disease did not experience any harmful consequences from eating gluten while they had hookworms in their intestines.

We don't suggest you start eating dirt or stop worming your pets, as you may acquire a harmful gut parasite that worsens your health problems. Instead, this highlights the significance of the gastrointestinal tract in autoimmune disease. You can get similar benefits from including probiotic rich foods such as fermented vegetables in your diet regularly. The good bacteria help to regulate and calm down an overactive immune system.

You can't prevent yourself from ever catching an infection. The types of infections linked with autoimmune disease are common infections that nearly everyone gets exposed to.

It is far more important to strengthen your immune system with a healthy diet and the right nutrients in order to overcome these infections

Chronic infections that linger in your body and continually irritate your immune system are the worst at triggering autoimmune disease.

Examples of common infections that can trigger autoimmune disease

Epstein-Barr virus (Glandular fever/mononucleosis)

This virus is in the herpes family of viruses and is an extremely common infection that just about everyone has suffered from at some point in their life. It's quite a sinister virus though; it is capable of triggering 33 different autoimmune diseases. Obviously not everyone who has had glandular fever goes on to develop 33 autoimmune diseases, let alone one. This virus is simply one of the known triggers. You also need to have the genetic susceptibility, an excessively permeable intestinal lining (leaky gut), nutrient deficiencies, stress and probably other factors as well.

The Epstein-Barr virus is most closely linked with the development of multiple sclerosis, systemic lupus erythematosus, rheumatoid arthritis and Sjogren's syndrome. Research has shown that some people with systemic lupus erythematosus have an elevated Epstein-Barr viral load in their bloodstream. It may be more than 15 times greater than in healthy individuals[8]. This means that some people are unable to clear the virus from their bloodstream because they have a weak immune system. The chronic stimulation of the immune system by the virus may go on for many years, and eventually lead to the development of an autoimmune disease.

Cytomegalovirus is also in the herpes family and it's a very common infection that approximately 40 percent of adults have had. Most people who get this virus don't get any symptoms, so they are completely unaware. If your immune system is weak, you may suffer with mild symptoms such as a sore throat, mild fever, swollen glands and a mildly swollen liver. Cytomegalovirus increases the risk of developing multiple sclerosis and Guillain Barre syndrome.

Helicobacter pylori

This the bacterium that increases the risk of stomach ulcers and stomach cancer. It is thought that more than half the world's population has this bacteria in their stomach, but most people do not develop symptoms or disease. If very high levels of Helicobacter pylori are present in the stomach, it can cause an inflamed stomach lining (gastritis) and symptoms of indigestion such as burping, bloating, nausea, stomach pain, reflux or heartburn.

There is a breath test, stool test and blood test for this bacteria. People who are treated for a stomach ulcer are typically given two different antibiotics, which are designed to kill this bug. That treatment is often not very effective; it either doesn't kill Helicobacter pylori adequately, or it does but the bacteria returns soon afterwards. Diet changes and nutritional supplements are usually more effective than antibiotics over the long term. It is important to improve the health of the digestive system, so it is no longer a hospitable environment for Helicobacter pylori.

Infection with this bacteria raises the risk of developing thrombocytopenia (low blood platelets), sarcoidosis, atherosclerosis, systemic sclerosis, antiphospholipid syndrome (can result in infertility), rheumatoid arthritis and psoriasis. Some research has shown that eradication of Helicobacter pylori can result in amelioration of autoimmune disease[9].

Streptococcal infections (Strep)

Streptococcal infections are very common. Strep throat is sometimes responsible for a sore throat, fever and enlarged lymph glands in the neck. The most common cause of a sore throat is a viral infection, while streptococcus is a type of bacteria. It is thought to be responsible for approximately 37 percent of cases of sore throat in children and only 5 to 15 percent in adults.

A small percentage of people who have had a strep infection go on to develop rheumatic fever, which is an autoimmune disease caused by antibody cross reactivity. The white blood cells had been producing antibodies against the strep bacteria, but for some reason the immune cells become confused and start making antibodies against the heart, skin, joints or brain. The surface molecules on the strep bacteria are so similar to some molecules of the human body, that a small percentage of people who get a strep infection go on to develop an autoimmune disease. Rheumatic fever can cause arthritis, myocarditis (inflammation of the heart), a skin rash and Sydenham chorea (a brain disease that causes involuntary movements of the face and arms).

Strep infections are also capable of triggering autoimmune kidney disease (glomerulonephritis), PANDAS (Pediatric Autoimmune Neuropsychiatric Disorders Associated with Streptococcal infections) and Tourette syndrome.

Chlamydia pneumoniae

This bacteria causes respiratory infections such as bronchitis, pharyngitis and pneumonia. It is not the same strain of bacteria that causes sexually transmitted infections. Infection with Chlamydia pneumoniae can increase the risk of Guillain Barre syndrome, arthritis, myocarditis, multiple sclerosis and Tourette syndrome. This can be a difficult infection to overcome because Chlamydia pneumoniae lives within human cells, therefore it is more resistant to treatment with antibiotics. Sticking to a healthy diet, as well as taking nutritional supplements such as vitamin D, Selenomune, zinc and vitamin C helps to overcome this infection.

Norovirus

Noroviruses are the most common cause of viral gastroenteritis (stomach flu). The most common symptoms of infection are vomiting, diarrhea, nausea and abdominal pain. Some people also experience a low grade fever, muscle aches and headaches. There is a strong relationship between infection with norovirus and subsequent development of Crohn's disease.

Hepatitis C

Infection with the hepatitis C virus is associated with a greater risk of developing the following autoimmune diseases: mixed cryoglobulinemia, systemic lupus erythematosus, Sjogren's syndrome and antiphospholipid syndrome.

Cell wall deficient bacteria (mycoplasma and chlamydia)

These organisms have a different structure to most other types of bacteria. Most bacteria require a cell wall in order to survive. Mycoplasma and chlamydia are able to survive without a cell wall because they are able to invade human cells. This makes the bacteria hard to detect and hard to treat. It also means they can cause long term, low grade, smouldering infections. The immune system often finds it very difficult to overcome these infections. The chronic immune stress caused by these infections increases the risk of autoimmune disease in genetically susceptible people.

Mycoplasma and chlamydia have been implicated in the development of several autoimmune diseases, as well as chronic fatigue syndrome, Gulf War syndrome and cancer. They can live within human cells and use your cell's DNA to replicate, just like viruses.

These organisms also seem to be capable of inducing molecular mimicry, meaning their structure mimics some of the protein fragments of human cells, thus encouraging the formation of auto-antibodies by your immune cells against your own body. Your immune system will detect the infection, but may find it very difficult to overcome. Your immune cells will produce inflammatory chemicals (cytokines), including tumour necrosis factor and interleukins, in an effort to fight these bugs. The chronic inflammation generated can cause fatigue, poor quality sleep, aches and pains and a low grade fever. The bacteria also release a lot of toxins into your body (called endotoxins), which further weaken your immune system and can even negatively affect your mood, emotions and cognitive abilities. In short, you'll feel rotten.

Most commonly used antibiotics kill bacteria by interfering with their ability to manufacture their cell wall. These types of antibiotics don't work on mycoplasma or chlamydia. Some clinicians recommend long term treatment (6 to 12 months) with several different antibiotics. Tetracycline and macrolide, as well as quinolone antibiotics, block the ability of mycoplasma and chlamydia to manufacture protein (so they won't be able to make DNA, thus can't survive).

Antibiotic regimes like this have been used successfully on victims of Gulf War illness, many of whom were found to be infected with a variety of different mycoplasma[10]. Research has also shown that treatment of these infections can offer dramatic health improvements in individuals with multiple sclerosis, systemic lupus erythematosus and chronic fatigue syndrome. However, it is controversial as to whether antibiotics can ever really permanently clear this type of infection, and there are definite risks and disadvantages associated with antibiotic use, particularly long term use. Therefore, we do not recommend antibiotics for most patients with these infections; certainly not as a first line therapy anyway.

The priority is to improve your diet, correct nutrient deficiencies, heal your gut and liver, and, in most instances, this will help your body to overcome these infections naturally

It is also difficult to get a mycoplasma infection accurately diagnosed. The standard pathology companies can test for only a few strains of mycoplasma, including pneumoniae and mycoplasma hominis, and mycoplasma genitalium, which can affect the genitourinary tract.

However, there are other mycoplasma infections. There are specialty laboratories that conduct PCR testing for these infections, which may be indicated for some people. PCR stands for Polymerase Chain Reaction and it is a test that checks for genetic material from a number of different bugs.

Chronic infections and autoimmune disease

Any persistent infections can also raise the risk of autoimmune disease in susceptible people. These are subtle, long term infections that may produce very few symptoms, therefore they typically go undetected and untreated. These infections can be bacterial, viral, parasitic or fungal. The infective agent can be present in your body in low numbers, therefore doesn't produce obvious symptoms. These infections can be hidden in various locations of the body, such as the sinuses, gums, bladder, gastrointestinal tract, uterus or other areas.

These infections can chronically stimulate your immune system, producing low grade inflammation. The toxins released by these bugs also weaken your immune system and can make you feel generally unwell. Common symptoms of low grade infections include fatigue, aches and pains, foggy head, low mood, poor quality sleep (particularly feeling too hot or alternating between feeling too hot and too cold), and unrefreshing sleep. Again, the most effective way to address these chronic infections is to strengthen your immune system.

Heavy metals

There is good evidence that heavy metals can trigger autoimmune disease, particularly aluminium, mercury, lead and gold. Exposure to toxic levels of heavy metals is very common in today's world and they come from a variety of sources.

Aluminium is a known neurotoxin that has long been implicated as a contributing factor to Alzheimer's disease. Just recently it is being linked to the development of autism. Aluminium is added to almost all vaccines and this represents the most significant source of aluminium exposure in children. Aluminium is added to vaccines because it behaves as an adjuvant (substance that elicits a strong immune response). In genetically susceptible individuals, this can trigger the development of an autoimmune disease.

Aluminium is also present in the following:

- Some deodorants and anti-perspirants
- Some cosmetics, moisturisers and toiletries
- Aluminium foil and cooking utensils
- Soft drink cans
- Some antacids contain aluminium

As mentioned, the greatest source of aluminium exposure for most people is through vaccines.

By the age of 5, if a child is given every vaccination in the current schedule, he/she will be exposed to nearly 15 times more aluminium than the FDA considers to be safe[11]

It's quite ironic to be giving vaccinations to a child to theoretically protect their health, while at the same time exposing them to exceedingly high levels of toxic substances.

Mercury adversely alters immune system function and increases the risk of autoimmune disease; particularly arthritis, lupus and thyroid disease[12]. Exposure to mercury prompts your immune system to produce more inflammatory chemicals and, if you are already genetically prone to getting an autoimmune disease, mercury toxicity can hasten the process. Mercury is added to the adult flu vaccine.

It is very important to try and minimise your exposure to this toxic metal. As well as causing immune system harm, mercury can also damage the brain and nervous system, impairing cognitive function and raising the risk of mood disorders.

The most common sources of mercury exposure include:

- Mercury dental amalgam fillings. These fillings contain inorganic mercury called ethylmercury. It is a more toxic form of this metal than the mercury found in some seafood. Mercury vapours are continually released from amalgam fillings, particularly old ones. If you have a large number of fillings in your mouth, or tests have shown you are suffering from mercury toxicity, you may want to consider having these fillings replaced. It is important to see a good holistic dentist who specialises in this procedure though, as the removal process can potentially expose you to far higher levels of mercury. Check that the dentist you wish to see is experienced at removing mercury amalgam fillings.

- Mercury has been taken out of most vaccines, however is still present in adult flu vaccines. Patients with an autoimmune disease are often advised to have the flu vaccine every year by their doctor because they are at increased risk of infection. This practice can expose you to dangerously high levels of mercury, as well as other toxins present in vaccines that adversely affect the immune system. The flu vaccine is a very controversial topic for several reasons. There has been great debate over whether it is even effective. In some patients it may cause more harm than good. Please discuss this matter with your own doctor, who can give you guidance on whether or not the flu vaccine is appropriate for you.

- Mercury is present in some seafood. Generally, large, long lived fish are the ones highest in mercury and other contaminants. Examples of fish that is fairly high in mercury and best avoided include swordfish, shark (flake), billfish, marlin, orange roughy, deep sea perch and catfish. Examples of fish lower in mercury include sardines, herrings, anchovies, mackerel and salmon. These species are also high in omega 3 fats, therefore are beneficial to include in your diet regularly. It is important to note that most fish is a fairly good source of the mineral selenium, and selenium helps to reduce mercury absorption by your body. If you are concerned about mercury exposure, we recommend you take a Selenomune in a dose of 150 to 200 mcg per day.

Gold has a long history of use for rheumatoid arthritis. It can help to relieve the pain and swelling of arthritis. However, gold can trigger other autoimmune diseases, particularly thrombocytopenia and immune complex mediated glomerulonephritis[13]. Wearing gold jewellery does not expose you to sufficiently high levels of gold to cause autoimmune disease. Cases of autoimmune disease generally occur from occupational exposure, such as in the mining industry.

Silicone

Silicone is another chemical that may trigger autoimmune disease. When most people think of silicone, they think of breast implants. This is certainly a very common use for silicone, but it is also used in medical tubing, as a component of joint replacements, and it is even used in cosmetic fillers that can be injected into your face to reduce the signs of ageing.

It was originally thought that silicone is an inert substance, with no effects on the immune system, but we now know that having silicone in your body can trigger a powerful immune response. Silicone increases proliferation of a type of immune cell called TH17 cells. These cells can create a great deal of inflammation and tissue damage in autoimmune disease.

Exposure to silicone has been associated with the following symptoms:

- Fatigue
- Weakness
- Muscle pain
- Joint pain
- Memory loss
- Loss of the protective myelin sheath around nerves due to destruction by antibodies[14].

Some women with breast implants develop a hard fibrous capsule around the implants, which is the immune system's way of isolating a foreign material that has entered the body and trying to protect the rest of your body from harm. This is one of the most common complications of silicone breast implant surgery. The collagen fiber capsule can thicken and compress the breast implant. This may be painful and could distort the shape of the breasts.

The most common autoimmune diseases associated with silicone exposure anywhere in the body include scleroderma, arthritis, multiple sclerosis and systemic lupus erythematosus. Silicone breast implants are big business, therefore there is quite some controversy over this topic and both industry and governments are inclined to deny these risks.

Interestingly, breast implants don't have to leak in order to trigger autoimmune disease

All breast implants diffuse small amounts of silicone into the bloodstream. If this persists for several years, and you have the genes for autoimmune disease, it may stimulate your immune system sufficiently to cause autoantibody production.

Does removal of breast implants lead to a cure of autoimmune disease? There have been reports of resolution of a disease following removal, however this is not the case in every patient. It seems to depend on how long the implants have been there, how much silicone has diffused out and how far it has travelled throughout the body.

Silicone can also be implanted or injected into the buttocks, to give them a rounder appearance. Implants carry the same risks as breast implants. Injections are far more harmful, but they are much cheaper, therefore very popular in some parts of the world. Silicone is a component of biopolymer injections, which have been linked to severe autoimmune diseases and even death.

The article below appeared in the American newspaper The Atlantic and highlights the problem in Venezuela very well.

Venezuelan Women are dying from Buttock Injections

The quest for beauty leads to a dangerous, DIY surgical procedure.

Alasdair Baverstock Sep 16, 2013

Astrid de la Rosa was left bedridden for two years after her liquid silicone buttock injections migrated into her spine, paralyzing the supporting muscles.

"We are trying to educate Venezuelan girls about the dangers of these procedures before they are 12 years old," she said. "We have to get to them early, as parents tend to offer these injections as 15th birthday presents".

In Venezuela, 17 women have died in the past 12 months as a result of liquid silicone buttock injections. The procedure, which according to Jesus Pereira, the president of the Veneuzelan Plastic Surgeons Association, an estimated 30 percent of Venezuelan women aged 18 to 50 have undergone, attempts to achieve a figure thought to be more attractive to Venezuelan men.

> *"When you live in a country where a beautiful woman has greater career prospects than someone with a strong work ethic, you are forced into the mindset that there is nothing more important than beauty."*

While the death toll resulting from these injections has risen since they became widely available in 2008, it has done little to curb the trend of Venezuelans seeking a quick-fix solution to what they perceive as physical inadequacies. Despite being illegal in Venezuela (sale of silicone carries a two-year prison sentence) the country's Association of Cosmetic Surgeons estimates that 2,000 women every month are receiving injections of this biopolymer, either at home or illegally at unlicensed businesses.

"The injections take just 20 minutes, but they can never fully be taken out," says Jesús Pereira, the president of the Venezuelan Plastic Surgeons Association. "100 percent of cases become complicated. It could take four days or it could take 20 years, but eventually the patient will become irreversibly sick."

Because the practice is banned, women seeking the procedure must find a fitness or beauty-related business that offers the injections in secret (most commonly a beauty salon or gym). The injections cost, on average, just $8.

The average Venezuelan woman spends 20 percent of her annual salary on beauty products, while 4,000 people go under the knife every month in the name of self-improvement.

Indeed, most banks in Venezuela offer long-term loan packages specifically tailored towards plastic surgery procedures.

Sadly, it has taken the death of one of the country's leading anti-biopolymer campaigners to awaken Venezuela to the dangers of these injections.

Mary Perdomo, the president and founder of the NO to Biopolymers, YES to Life foundation, died several weeks ago as a result of the buttock injections she received four years ago. The mother of three had used her worsening illness as a method to teach fellow Venezuelans about the fatal risks the phenomenon poses.

In 2009, Perdomo underwent the standard procedure of having 560cc of the poisonous biopolymer injected into each cheek. Three months later she began to have trouble sleeping and later discovered tumors that had formed in the affected area. In 2012, the health campaigner was diagnosed with an autoimmune disease: a direct result of her body's reaction to the foreign chemicals. She died earlier this month following a heart attack.

Perdomo's legacy lives on through the various organizations that work to educate young Venezuelans about biopolymers.

"For the past three years I've been on a daily cocktail of painkillers and antibiotics, it's the only way I can live with the pain," says Astrid de la Rosa, who uses herself as an example as she tours middle schools in the Caracas area.

"More than the physical agony, I was psychologically damaged by what happened to me," she said. "When the rashes and fevers began, my partner left me, and I was left alone with a 4-year-old child whom I couldn't support because I couldn't physically work".

De la Rosa, along with the NO to Biopolymers foundation, claims the government needs to work harder to educate young Venezuelans about the dangers of liquid silicone, and fight to stop the procedure, which is now classified as a "public health issue," from being offered in the first place.

"Lamentably, the majority of the people receiving these injections are young women from poorer backgrounds who haven't been educated to the enormous risks that these injections pose," Pereira said. "They feel put under pressure by friends or society, and look for quick solutions."

Despite Venezuelan law imposing strict sanctions over the handling of biopolymers, state regulation here is minimal. Those who wish to conduct the procedure themselves need only to source the biopolymer through Internet vendors, a very simple task, as I discovered when I did a quick search for a 500cc bottle myself.

"It's very simple," said Omaira, an internet vendor who asked her last name not be used. Omaira advertises her wares on the Latin American second-hand market website mercadolibre.com "You have to transfer the 350 Bolívars ($8.50) into my bank account, and I'll send someone out to deliver them."

"What we do is completely illegal, so you can't come to the place where we stock the substance," she said. "But we've never had any problems with the police, nor has anyone who has ever bought this product from us".

It is perhaps unsurprising that biopolymer-related illness is on the rise in Venezuela. These injections are the latest in a long list of extreme beauty procedures in this beauty-obsessed country. Other extreme self-improvement methods include fasting pacts among friends, vomit-inducing syrup, and most recently the sewing of a plastic patch onto the tongue, which renders the consumption of solid food extremely painful.

Venezuela's beauty trade is worth an annual average of $2.5 billion dollars in a nation whose population is just 29 million. Only petroleum is more profitable.

The country also has a reputation for beautiful women -- it holds the Guinness World Record for the nation with the most international beauty queens. "Las Miss" (The Misses) as they are known in Venezuela go on to profitable careers. In 1998, former Venezuelan Miss Universe Irene Saez unsuccessfully ran against Hugo Chavez for the country's presidency.

"Every girl here dreams of being a Miss. We Venezuelans see those people as the perfect women," says Maria Trinidad, a representative of the NO to Biopolymers foundation who sold her car in order to pay for an invasive surgery to remove her injections.

"When you live in a country where a beautiful woman has greater career prospects than someone with a strong work ethic and first-class education, you are forced into the mindset that there is nothing more important than beauty."

"To be 'operada' (to have undergone plastic surgery) is completely normal in Venezuela," says Oriana Gonzalez, who paid for her own breast enhancements at age 20 over the protestations of her parents. "It's simply not viewed as extreme in the way that other cultures perceive it."

As a result of this more open mindset toward surgically enhanced physicality, Venezuela has garnered an international reputation as an inexpensive and safe destination for plastic surgery. While the average price for silicone implants in the United States is $8,000, the same procedure in the South American nation costs just $800.

"Education is the key," said De la Rosa. "If we can teach the next generations that these quick-fix solutions to looking our best aren't actually solutions at all, then we have a better chance."

"As for Venezuelan men, they shouldn't worry," she says. "We're still the most beautiful women in the world."

www.theatlantic.com/international/archive/2013/09/venezuelan-women-are-dying-from-buttock-injections/279693/?single_page=true

Vaccinations

The issue of autoimmune disease being triggered by vaccinations is a very controversial topic, however there are many well documented cases of specific autoimmune diseases resulting from specific vaccinations. There are several different components of a vaccine that can harm the immune system:

- The infective agent. Vaccines use a modified form of a virus or bacterium that is no longer capable of causing an infection, but is capable of eliciting an immune response and antibody production. Fragments of the virus or bacterium may resemble components of our own body and through a process called molecular mimicry, may trigger the production of antibodies against your own body.

- Adjuvants. The word adjuvant means to assist. Every vaccine requires an adjuvant in order to wake up the immune system and prompt it to manufacture antibodies. Adjuvants are often referred to as "the immunologists dirty little trick" in medical journals because they are present in all vaccines in order to make them more effective, but most people don't know about them[15].

- The most commonly used adjuvants include mercury, aluminium, squalene, mineral oils (petroleum derived), silicone, viral particles and Freund's adjuvant (the name of a person who developed a combination of mineral oil with bacterial particles).

- Mercury was removed from most vaccines apart from the adult flu vaccine. It has largely been replaced with aluminium because it is cheap and doesn't have as bad publicity as mercury. It's still toxic in high doses, of course.

- Preservatives and stabilisers. A range of different chemicals are added to maintain the integrity of the vaccine.

- Culture medium. Most of the vaccines in use today are grown in a culture of yeast. The yeast is called Sarrharomyces cerevisiae.

This is the same type of yeast that is used for baking and brewing. The yeast is not harmful to most people but allergies to it are very common, particularly among people with autoimmune disease, especially lupus.

The potential dangers of childhood vaccinations

Injecting these toxic substances into the bloodstream of any person is risky, but the dangers are greatly multiplied in children. This is because of their smaller body size, less developed detoxification capabilities and the large number of vaccinations given in a very short space of time.

The following passage is an excerpt from a research paper published in the journal, Lupus. The paper is titled *Mechanisms of aluminum adjuvant toxicity and autoimmunity in pediatric populations:*

"Immune challenges during early development, including those vaccine-induced, can lead to permanent detrimental alterations of the brain and immune function. Experimental evidence also shows that simultaneous administration of as little as two to three immune adjuvants can overcome genetic resistance to autoimmunity.

In some developed countries, by the time children are 4 to 6 years old, they will have received a total of 126 antigenic compounds along with high amounts of aluminum (Al) adjuvants through routine vaccinations.

According to the US Food and Drug Administration, safety assessments for vaccines have often not included appropriate toxicity studies because vaccines have not been viewed as inherently toxic. Taken together, these observations raise plausible concerns about the overall safety of current childhood vaccination programs.

When assessing adjuvant toxicity in children, several key points ought to be considered:

(i)   infants and children should not be viewed as "small adults" with regard to toxicological risk as their unique physiology makes them much more vulnerable to toxic insults;

(ii) in adult humans Al vaccine adjuvants have been linked to a variety of serious autoimmune and inflammatory conditions (i.e., "Autoimmune Syndrome Induced by Adjuvants"), yet children are regularly exposed to much higher amounts of Al from vaccines than adults;

(iii) it is often assumed that peripheral immune responses do not affect brain function.

However, it is now clearly established that there is a bidirectional neuro-immune cross-talk that plays crucial roles in immuno-regulation as well as brain function. In turn, perturbations of the neuro-immune axis have been demonstrated in many autoimmune diseases encompassed in "ASIA" and are thought to be driven by a hyperactive immune response; and

(iv) the same components of the neuro-immune axis that play key roles in brain development and immune function are heavily targeted by Al adjuvants.

In summary, research evidence shows that increasing concerns about current vaccination practices may indeed be warranted. Because children may be most at risk of vaccine-induced complications, a rigorous evaluation of the vaccine-related adverse health impacts in the pediatric population is urgently needed."[16]

This is not a book about vaccinations. A great deal has been written about this subject by other authors. We merely want to point out that there's a strong relationship between vaccinations and the onset of autoimmune disease. If you have children and you or their other parent have autoimmune disease, you may wish to delay and stagger the vaccinations they are given, in order to reduce exposure to toxic chemicals that may harm their immune system at such a critical time in their development.

Examples of autoimmune diseases triggered by vaccinations

The autoimmune disease with the strongest links to vaccination is Guillain Barre syndrome. This is a disease that affects the peripheral nervous system (the central nervous system refers to the brain and spinal cord). The most common symptoms are weakness in the arms and legs and sometimes a feeling of being paralysed.

The flu vaccine

There have been several documented cases of individuals developing Guillian-Barre syndrome following the flu vaccination. In 1976, after a US government sponsored mass vaccination program in which 45 million adults received the flu vaccine, there was a 4 to 8 times greater incidence of Guillian-Barre syndrome. It is not a very common disease, therefore the sharp rise in incidence was highly significant. This incident was reported in the New England Journal of Medicine.[17]

Narcolepsy is an autoimmune disease that causes a person to involuntarily fall asleep during waking hours. Sometimes it is accompanied by cataplexy, where they also lose a great deal of muscle strength and may fall to the ground. In August 2010, neurologists from Sweden and Finland reported a 13 fold higher incidence of narcolepsy among children aged between 4 and 19 years, who had received the H1N1 flu vaccine. Symptoms of the disease appeared within days to 6 months, with the average being 2.5 months[18]. Narcolepsy is a serious disease and not a common disease, therefore this strong association with the flu vaccine has concerned many researchers.

Hepatitis B vaccine

There is growing concern over the safety and the effectiveness of the hepatitis B vaccine. A study published in the Journal of the American Medical Association (JAMA) titled "Hair loss after routine immunizations" reported an increased risk of alopecia areata following vaccination for hepatitis B[19]. Alopecia areata is hair loss that occurs all over the body; scalp hair is lost, as well as all body hair. Mild cases typically cause bald patches on the scalp.

Other studies have shown an increased risk of multiple sclerosis following vaccination. There was a threefold increase in the incidence of multiple sclerosis in the three years following vaccination for hepatitis B[20].

It is interesting to note that studies have shown people with celiac disease are poor responders to the hepatitis B vaccination. Research has shown that between 4 and 10 percent of healthy individuals do not respond to the hepatitis B vaccine. This means they don't produce sufficient antibodies to provide immunity from disease. Among celiacs, approximately 61 percent do not respond to the vaccination[21]. This is thought to be due to genetic factors.

Individuals who already have an autoimmune disease are more at risk of developing a second or third autoimmune disease, and vaccinations are one known trigger. It's interesting then to consider that celiacs may be more prone to harm caused by the vaccine, while being less likely to experience the benefits.

Autoimmune disease in vaccinated farmed salmon

Even salmon can develop autoimmune disease after being vaccinated! Most of the salmon produced in the world today is farmed. It's a lot more economical for salmon producers that way. However, living in cramped conditions and not being able to feed on their natural diet has made the salmon prone to disease. One of the strategies used to manage this problem is vaccination.

Interestingly enough, it didn't take long for health problems to develop in the salmon. Laboratory testing revealed the presence of auto-antibodies in the bloodstream. X-rays have revealed inflammatory damage and granulomas in several organs[22]. Yes, the researchers actually went to the trouble of X-raying the salmon!

Bisphenol A (BPA)

Bisphenol A is a chemical used in the manufacture of polycarbonate plastic. It is present in a wide range of commonly used items such as plastic containers, utensils, toys, water bottles, the inner lining of some food cans, plastic lids of disposable coffee cups (and the inner lining of paper coffee cups); and it is even found in sales receipts. BPA has been shown to leach out of products, and high levels have been identified in human tissue samples. In fact, research has shown that more than 90 percent of the US population has detectable levels in their urine.

Heat and acidic substances increase the leaching of BPA into foods; therefore it's best to avoid drinking hot coffee or tea out of disposable cups, and eating canned tomatoes (acidic) from BPA lined cans. You would have noticed a great number of plastic items labelled BPA free in recent years. That's nothing to get excited about, as research has shown the BPA substitutes are just as bad. Bisphenol S is the most widely used substitute and it too appears to have adverse health effects.

It has been known for a long time that bisphenol A is an endocrine disruptor. That means it disrupts the hormone balance in the body. It has particularly adverse effects on the sex hormones (estrogen and testosterone), as well as thyroid hormones. Very recent studies have shown that BPA affects the immune system in a number of harmful ways, and may raise the risk of developing an autoimmune disease, or aggravating an existing disease. Specifically, it stimulates production of the same inflammatory immune chemicals that other environmental toxins such as silicone and vaccinations induce[23].

At this stage, there is no research linking bisphenol A to specific autoimmune diseases. If you have an autoimmune disease, it is best to limit your exposure to plastic as much as possible. Try to store food and water in glass or stainless steel containers, and especially avoid heating foods or liquids in plastic containers.

Cigarettes

Most people don't associate smoking cigarettes with the development of autoimmune disease, however smokers are more likely to develop rheumatoid arthritis, lupus, inflammatory bowel disease and Graves' disease. Smoking changes the structure of some proteins in the lungs, which your immune system then won't recognise as your own. In some genetically predisposed individuals, this can cause the development of Goodpasture syndrome. This is a rare but serious disease that can cause bleeding in the lungs, as well as kidney failure.

Smokers tend to respond poorly to treatment for their autoimmune disease compared to non-smokers.

Drugs/medication

There are several medications that can trigger autoimmune disease in genetically susceptible people. The most well known case is drug induced lupus, however autoimmune hepatitis, ulcerative colitis and other autoimmune diseases may be triggered by drugs. The most likely culprits include antibiotics (particularly isoniazid, Nitrofurantoin, Minocycline), hydralazine (used for high blood pressure), isotretinoin (used for acne) and procainamide (used for abnormal heart rhythms) and anticonvulsants, used for epilepsy. In some cases, stopping the medication can ameliorate the autoimmune disease but people who develop drug induced autoimmune disease were already genetically susceptible, and may have even had a mild subclinical form of the disease, which was just unmasked by the drug.

Stress

Intense stress or long term stress has an extremely harmful effect on the immune system. Many people associate the beginning of their autoimmune disease with a stressful life incident. Stress is never the sole factor responsible for the development of a disease though; rather it just promotes the start of something you were prone to getting anyway. A stressful life episode may trigger the initial development of an autoimmune disease, and it is a common cause of a flare up in people living with autoimmune disease.

It also needs to be mentioned that having an autoimmune disease can be a significant source of stress in your life. It is common to feel frightened, overwhelmed and alone at times, because severe fatigue and or pain can make coping with day to day challenges extremely difficult.

> *Your family and friends may not be able to understand the overwhelming fatigue you experience and this can feel quite isolating*

Unfortunately, stress can be a major block to recovery. If there is a major ongoing source of stress in your life it may be very difficult to achieve a significant improvement in your health until the stress abates.

The stress hormones that your body manufactures when you are upset promote your immune system to produce more inflammatory cytokines. These chemicals heighten immune activation in your body and make autoimmune disease more likely or more intense.

Exercise that is too intense or of too long duration can also act like a stress to your body by promoting high cortisol secretion. Exercise is very important but if you're chronically stressed, sleeping poorly, suffering a great deal of fatigue or pain, it is best to stick to mild forms of exercise that do not overexert your body. It is also best to not exercise for longer than 30 minutes at a time, as this will also help to prevent the exercise from being overly stressful to your body.

The main stress hormones in your body are adrenalin and cortisol. We will focus on cortisol because it has greater effects on the immune system than adrenalin. Cortisol is made from cholesterol in your adrenal glands. Interestingly, it shares a metabolic pathway with progesterone production, therefore chronic stress in women can cause cortisol excess and progesterone deficiency. Progesterone deficiency can cause menstrual problems and raises the risk of conditions such as endometriosis and uterine fibroids.

Cortisol is involved in the fight or flight acute stress response, but it is also released if you suffer with chronic stress. Being stressed for a long time can cause you to have chronically elevated cortisol levels.

Chronically elevated cortisol can have a negative effect on your blood sugar level; it may raise your blood sugar and promote abdominal weight gain. Elevated cortisol can worsen insulin resistance (syndrome X) and eventually put you at increased risk of type 2 diabetes. Cortisol's effects on your blood sugar tend to encourage sugar and carbohydrate cravings. Therefore if you've been feeling stressed out, you're more likely to crave sugar and high carb foods. Chronically elevated cortisol also weakens the immune system and makes you more prone to coming down with infections.

Cortisol has negative effects on the digestive tract. It opens up the tight junctions between intestinal cells and promotes leaky gut syndrome. This has a major negative burden on the immune system and is discussed in great detail in chapter 4.

Long term stress can give you chronically elevated cortisol, but it's not just emotional stress that may be responsible. Don't forget that illness is a major stress on the body and autoimmune disease definitely takes its toll.

Unhealthy food also stresses your adrenal glands, and food intolerance can have the same effect

The eating plan in chapter six excludes the most common offenders.

Long term problems with the adrenal glands can lead to adrenal gland exhaustion. This can impede healing and worsen pain and fatigue. It is covered in detail in chapter eight.

Female hormones and pregnancy

Approximately three quarters of patients with autoimmune disease are women, and women are at higher risk of developing an autoimmune disease following childbirth; therefore female hormones must play an important role. Some autoimmune diseases fluctuate in intensity throughout the month, depending on the phase of a woman's menstrual cycle. Some autoimmune diseases go into remission during pregnancy, while others intensify markedly.

Estrogen and progesterone are the main female sex hormones. Women also produce male hormones (called androgens), such as testosterone, albeit in much lower quantities than men. Estrogen is predominantly produced during the first half of the menstrual cycle. It stimulates thickening of the endometrium, preparing it for pregnancy. Progesterone is produced in the second half of the menstrual cycle, following ovulation.

Estrogen tends to have a bad reputation because in some situations it can promote the development of endometriosis, uterine fibroids, painful breasts, heavy menstrual bleeding, breast cancer and PMS. An imbalance between estrogen and progesterone is extremely common and this is known as estrogen dominance. There is too little progesterone in relation to estrogen. Any medical condition that inhibits ovulation will also produce a progesterone deficiency. Polycystic ovarian syndrome is the most common example. Stress can also inhibit ovulation, and the lack of ovulation can aggravate an existing autoimmune disease.

The sex hormones are known as steroid hormones because they have a steroid like structure and are closely related to cholesterol and cortisol. Steroids are commonly given to patients with autoimmune disease because they reduce inflammation. Prednisone is the most common example.

Steroid hormones have anti-inflammatory effects and this is also true for progesterone. This is not surprising when you consider that progesterone and cortisol are both manufactured from cholesterol, and progesterone is just one step further down the production chain. The following diagram explains hormone production well.

How cholesterol is converted into steroid hormones

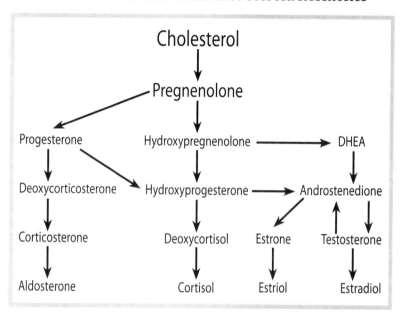

Women with autoimmune disease commonly experience an aggravation or flare in the second half of their menstrual cycle if they are not producing adequate progesterone. This can be ameliorated well with the use of a natural bio-identical progesterone cream. You can also support progesterone production by ensuring your diet contains sufficient vitamins and minerals and healthy fats (since progesterone is mostly made of fat). However, if you have an autoimmune disease and are low in progesterone, you should experience faster improvements in your wellbeing with a bio-identical progesterone cream. This cream requires a doctor's prescription.

Symptoms of progesterone deficiency

If you are suffering with an autoimmune disease and you experience several of the following symptoms, you may benefit from progesterone:

- Heavy menstrual bleeding
- Painful periods, especially if the pain lasts more than 24 hours
- Irregular menstrual periods
- Endometriosis
- Uterine fibroids
- Adenomyosis (thickening of the uterine muscle)
- Endometrial hyperplasia (excessively thick uterine lining)
- Premenstrual syndrome (PMS)
- Polycystic ovarian syndrome (PCOS)
- Postnatal depression
- Scalp hair loss or thinning
- Breast pain or lumpy breasts
- Insomnia in the week before menstruation

Other hormone deficiencies

People with autoimmune disease often suffer with low levels of certain hormones. Low levels of adrenal gland hormones are common in people with adrenal gland exhaustion. We often discover low levels of the hormone DHEA (dehydroepiandrosterone), and sometimes the patient greatly benefits from the prescription of bio-identical DHEA. This is discussed in more detail on page 201.

Pregnenolone

Pregnenolone is a steroid hormone made in your body from cholesterol. It is considered a mother hormone because your body uses it to produce a large range of other hormones. It can be used to produce progesterone, androgens (male hormones), estrogen and hormones made by the adrenal glands. Pregnenolone helps to reduce inflammation in your body. It has similar actions to cortisol.

Long term illness, stress, exhaustion and nutrient deficiencies can create a deficiency in this hormone, and this is typical in autoimmune patients. Taking pregnenolone in supplement form can help to reduce aches and pains and improve energy and stamina. It has many of the benefits of steroids such as prednisone, without the harmful side effects, as long as it's used in an appropriate dose. Pregnenolone requires a doctor's prescription and needs to be made by a compounding pharmacy.

Estriol

Estriol is a type of estrogen. Women actually produce three different types of estrogen in their bodies: estriol, oestrone and oestradiol. Estriol is the mildest form. Some women with autoimmune disease suffer with prematurely low levels of estrogen, and supplementing with this hormone can offer improvements for some conditions.

Research conducted on women with multiple sclerosis showed that taking estriol can reduce the risk of flare ups of the disease[24]. This is because estriol is able to reach the brain and protect brain cells from damage. Multiple sclerosis is one of those autoimmune diseases that usually improves significantly while a woman is pregnant, and then worsens after she gives birth. This is partly because estrogen (and progesterone) levels become very high during pregnancy. Taking a small amount of estriol and progesterone long term may offer women some of these benefits. Estriol requires a doctor's prescription.

Postpartum autoimmune disease

Postpartum means after delivering a child. Quite commonly, an autoimmune disease will first appear following childbirth. The most common autoimmune diseases to develop after giving birth are postpartum thyroiditis and postpartum autoimmune hepatitis.

Postpartum thyroiditis

Postpartum thyroiditis is inflammation of the thyroid gland that occurs in five to nine percent of women during the first six months after giving birth. The thyroid gland can become enlarged but this is usually not painful.

Symptoms of postpartum thyroiditis

There are usually two phases to this disease: first hyperthyroidism, then hypothyroidism. In the first phase, while the thyroid gland is inflamed it releases too much hormone into the bloodstream. This phase usually lasts two to four months and it causes the metabolism to speed up. Women commonly experience the symptoms of hyperthyroidism such as: weight loss, a rapid heart rate, anxiety, increased sweating and sensitivity to heat. These symptoms are usually quite mild and many women barely notice them.

In the second phase, the thyroid gland does not produce enough hormones, and this causes the symptoms of hypothyroidism. This phase can last up to a year. Some women develop a goitre (enlarged thyroid gland); other symptoms can include: depression, fatigue, sensitivity to cold, constipation, dry skin and brittle nails, weight gain and hair loss. The condition can be diagnosed by measuring levels of the hormones TSH, T3 and T4 in the blood, as well as thyroid antibodies.

What causes postpartum thyroiditis?

The condition is an autoimmune disease. The body's immune system incorrectly identifies the thyroid gland as a foreign invader and produces antibodies to destroy it. While women are pregnant, their immune system becomes somewhat suppressed so that they don't produce antibodies that could harm the developing foetus. This is partly due to high levels of progesterone during pregnancy. After delivery, the immune system becomes reactivated again. It is during this time that the thyroid gland can become inflamed from postpartum thyroiditis.

Some women have thyroid antibodies in their bloodstream while pregnant and approximately 30 to 50 percent of them will go on to develop postpartum thyroiditis.

Women with the following conditions are most at risk of developing postpartum thyroiditis:

- High levels of antithyroid antibodies during the first trimester of pregnancy.

- An immune system disorder or autoimmune disease, such as type 1 diabetes, rheumatoid arthritis, celiac disease or lupus. Women with type 1 diabetes are three times more likely to develop postpartum thyroiditis than non-diabetic women.

- A personal or family history of thyroid disease, for example Graves' disease or Hashimoto's thyroiditis.

- Goitre (enlarged thyroid gland).

- A history of postpartum thyroiditis. Women who have had this condition with one pregnancy have a 20 percent chance of being affected in subsequent pregnancies.

Women with antithyroid antibodies in their bloodstream are at increased risk of infertility, miscarriage and postpartum depression.

Treatment of postpartum thyroiditis

In the first phase, when the thyroid gland produces excessive levels of hormones, symptoms are often mild and require no treatment. If tremors and a rapid heart rate are present, beta blocker drugs can be given for a short time to relieve these symptoms. During the second phase, when the thyroid cannot produce adequate hormones, thyroxine (T4) hormone replacement is usually given to restore normal hormone levels. Very little of the prescribed thyroid hormone passes through the placenta to the foetus, or into breast milk. It is safe to use while pregnant or breastfeeding. Suffering from untreated hypothyroidism while pregnant or breastfeeding can have dangerous consequences to the intellectual development of a newborn baby.

Most women take prescription thyroxine tablets for approximately six months. After that time, the patient will be told to stop the tablets for four to six weeks and have a blood test for TSH, T4 and T3 hormones. This lets us know if the hypothyroidism is permanent, or if the thyroid has recovered and can now produce its own thyroid hormones again. Around 25 to 30 percent of women are left with permanent hypothyroidism and they must take prescribed thyroid hormone replacement for life.

All women who have had postpartum thyroiditis are at increased risk of developing Hashimoto's thyroiditis later in life, or another autoimmune disease.

Minimising the risks of postpartum thyroiditis

After giving birth, many women experience several months of exhaustion and emotional upheavals. Many women also experience postnatal depression and this can become very debilitating if not recognised and treated. It is very important to have your thyroid function tested regularly by your doctor because postpartum thyroiditis is easily treated and it may be causing you unnecessary suffering.

If you are planning pregnancy, make sure you ask your doctor to do a blood test for antithyroid antibodies and TSH; especially if you:

- Have an autoimmune disease. In particular type 1 diabetes, but also rheumatoid arthritis, lupus, celiac disease and others.
- Have a goitre.
- Have a thyroid disease.
- Have a strong family history of thyroid disease.
- Have had postpartum thyroiditis before.

Nutritional deficiencies

Being deficient in certain critical nutrients can raise your risk of autoimmune disease. Nutrient deficiencies are very common among Americans, and in fact in most places around the world. Modern food has become quick, tasty and convenient, while food quality has been declining.

Even if you are very careful about the type of food you eat, and mostly avoid processed foods, nutrient levels in the soil in many parts of the USA have been falling, therefore the foods will be lacking certain nutrients. Fruits and vegetables bought from the supermarket have often been in storage for many months, or may have been frozen. Nutrients in fresh produce start to deteriorate as soon as they're picked from the tree or pulled from the soil.

This is a good reason to support your local farmers' market. Even if the produce is not organic, at least it was grown locally and you're buying it soon after harvest (often it was only picked from the ground the day before). You'll probably also notice that fruit and vegetables you've bought from a local farmers' market remain fresh and crisp a lot longer than those purchased from a supermarket.

Perhaps you could grow some fresh produce in your own backyard. Herbs and leafy vegetables such as silverbeet and kale are particularly easy to grow and don't require much space at all. If you live in an apartment or can't use the soil in your own backyard, perhaps you could grow some herbs in pots.

Nothing beats the flavor and freshness of home grown produce, and you'll know it's free of chemical sprays or artificial fertilisers

Optimum levels of nutrients are required for healthy immune system function; to help reduce the risk of both infections and autoimmune disease. Commonly, the diet will be deficient in vitamins and minerals, while at the same time contain an excess of sugar, artificial food additives and omega 6 rich industrial seed oils. This sets the stage for chronic high levels of inflammation in the body.

Modern diets are typically deficient in healthy fats. This is because the average person tries to avoid oily or fatty foods, thinking they are unhealthy, or that they'll cause weight gain. Nothing could be further from the truth. Healthy fats are critical for a healthy metabolism, and satiety, and when consumed in the context of a lower carbohydrate diet, can actually promote weight loss. Foods high in healthy fats are often a source of fat soluble vitamins, and fats are necessary for the absorption of fat soluble vitamins, plus many different antioxidants.

In modern diets, factory processed seed oils, such as canola oil, cottonseed oil, soybean oil and sunflower oil have largely replaced traditional fats such as butter, lard and coconut oil. The industrial seed oils are very high in omega 6 fats and they skew the optimal ratio between omega 6 and omega 3 fats. In general, an excess of some omega 6 fats can increase inflammation while omega 3 fats lower it. Grain fed meat, chicken and eggs are fairly high in omega 6 fats, while grass fed (pasture raised) animals are higher in omega 3 fats.

The types of healthy fats we're referring to include extra virgin olive oil, avocados, oily fish, coconut oil and the fat on grass fed meat. There is more information about the beneficial effects of fats in chapter six.

Healthy diet, yet still nutrient deficient?

A common problem among people with autoimmune disease is poor nutrient absorption. You could be eating a fantastic diet, yet not absorbing the nutrients well. The end result is you won't be much better off than the people who don't care about their diet and eat any type of junk food that takes their fancy. It's certainly not fair but it often happens.

The typical autoimmune patient has weak digestion. They have low levels of stomach acid and pancreatic enzymes, and a poorly functioning liver, therefore inadequate bile. Gluten intolerance or other food sensitivities can inflame the intestinal lining, creating leaky gut syndrome. Small Intestinal Bacterial Overgrowth (SIBO) can also inflame the gut lining, compromising nutrient absorption.

Leaky gut allows the entry of wastes in the intestines into the bloodstream, but it also hinders the proper absorption of important vitamins, minerals and other nutrients. Healing leaky gut and restoring digestive health is the key to improving immune and liver health. See chapter four for our recommendations on how to achieve that.

Many people believe they are following a healthy diet and eating healthy food because they're listening to conventional dietary advice, which encourages the consumption of grains and low fat dairy products. These foods are difficult to digest for many; provide very few nutrients in your diet and can actually rob your body of nutrients. Grains look like healthy foods on paper; they are a source of B vitamins and minerals such as magnesium and zinc. However, grains also contain substances that bind with minerals and inhibit their absorption, as well as substances that irritate the gut lining, promoting leaky gut syndrome. We go into detail about the problem with grains in chapter five. Some people are able to tolerate grains well; they can consume them and maintain a great level of health. People with autoimmune disease usually don't fall into that category.

The table below has been adapted from the paper Origins and evolution of the Western diet: health implications for the 21st century, published in the American Journal of Clinical Nutrition. You can see that the most nutrient dense foods are vegetables, followed by meat and seafood, then fruit and so on. There are no nutrients present in grains, legumes and dairy products that you can't obtain from other foods.

If you base your diet on vegetables, fruit, animal protein, nuts and healthy fats, you'll be getting plenty of nutrients and won't risk nutritional deficiencies. This is especially true if you eat offal, bone broth and fermented vegetables. So there really isn't any need to worry about suffering nutrient deficiencies if you're cutting out entire food groups (grains, legumes and dairy products). In fact, once you heal your intestines you'll be absorbing far more nutrients from the foods you're eating than what you are probably absorbing now.

As you can see in the table, whole milk is a good source of nutrients, but its disadvantages greatly outweigh its advantages for anyone with autoimmune disease, therefore we recommend you avoid it.

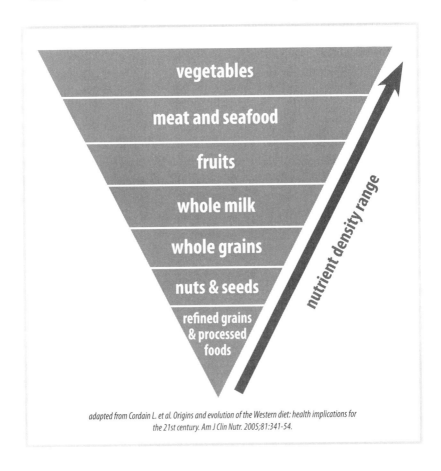

adapted from Cordain L. et al. Origins and evolution of the Western diet: health implications for the 21st century. Am J Clin Nutr. 2005;81:341-54.

Vitamin D insufficiency and autoimmune disease

Even if you live in a sunny country, you may not have enough vitamin D in your bloodstream. This is a problem because it places a person at higher risk of developing an autoimmune disease, and if you already have one, it will make the disease more severe and raise the risk of flares. Vitamin D can reduce or halt the production of auto-antibodies. This means it may be capable of arresting an autoimmune disease. See chaper seven for more information about vitamin D and other nutrients necessary for reversing autoimmune disease.

Selenium and autoimmune disease

Selenium is very important for a healthy immune system and it is beneficial for all types of autoimmune disease. However, there is a particularly strong relationship between selenium and the thyroid gland. Hashimoto's thyroiditis is the most common autoimmune disease in the world. It occurs when the immune system produces antibodies directed at the thyroid gland. Over time, these antibodies inflame the thyroid and reduce its ability to manufacture hormones. Eventually the thyroid gland becomes underactive and hypothyroidism is diagnosed.

The soils of many parts of the world are notoriously low in selenium, and this includes many parts of the USA.

Therefore most foods are not a good source of this mineral, with the exception of Brazil nuts. Many farmers give selenium supplements to their cattle because they know the soil contains insufficient levels, and therefore the grass and grains won't contain enough. People with poor digestion or a digestive disease such as celiac disease or inflammatory bowel disease are much more prone to selenium deficiency than the general population.

There is more information about selenium in chapter seven.

Food sensitivities

Hidden food sensitivities raise your risk of developing an autoimmune disease because they inflame your intestines, creating leaky gut syndrome, and they chronically over stimulate your immune system.

Food sensitivities encompass food allergies and food intolerance. Food intolerance is far more common and more difficult to uncover. Food allergies typically produce immediate and severe symptoms, such as hives, a skin rash, breathing difficulties or full blown anaphylactic shock. The offending food or foods are usually promptly detected and an individual learns to steer clear of them.

The scenario is usually quite different with food intolerance because the symptoms are more subtle and less immediate. The symptoms of food intolerance can first appear anywhere from one to three days after you've ingested the food. The symptoms can also be so vague and broad that you'd never suspect to link them to what you've eaten. The foods most likely to trigger an intolerance are usually commonly eaten items that most people consume at least once each day.

Food sensitivity is a problem because it causes inflammation in your body, and inflammation is a major driver of autoimmune disease. The gut lining is the major target of inflammation, and research has shown that an inflamed gut is the biggest predisposing factor in developing autoimmune disease. You will not be able to heal leaky gut syndrome if you continue to consume a food you are sensitive to.

Once the lining of the gut is inflamed, your ability to absorb nutrients is impaired, while at the same time you'll be absorbing things that are supposed to stay in your gut. These things include bacteria and other microbes, bacterial toxins and incompletely digested foods. Absorbing incompletely digested foods sets the stage for the development of new food sensitivities. It can be a vicious cycle, where more and more foods are making you unwell. The way to resolve this problem is to identify problematic foods, remove them from your diet and work on healing a leaky gut.

Symptoms of food sensitivities

The following list describes possible symptoms:

Respiratory system: asthma, hay fever, runny nose (rhinitis), post-nasal drip (mucus running down the back of the throat), blocked nose, particularly at night, chronic cough, sore throat or itchy throat.

Ears and eyes: blocked ears, repeated ear infections, red ears, particularly after a meal, runny eyes, conjunctivitis, sensitivity to light, gritty or itchy eyes, eczema on or around the eyes.

Digestive system: diarrhea, constipation, irritable bowel syndrome, abdominal bloating, flatulence, burping, abdominal cramps, heartburn, reflux, nausea, indigestion.

Urinary system: frequent night time urination, urinary incontinence, weak bladder, interstitial cystitis.

Emotional: anxiety, depression, fatigue, particularly after meals, poor concentration, restlessness, insomnia or frequent night time waking, hyperactivity.

Muscular and skeletal: joint pain, muscle aches, muscle cramps, weak muscles.

Skin: eczema, dermatitis, hives, flushed cheeks, itchy skin, dandruff, dark rings under the eyes.

Miscellaneous: Low grade fever, night time perspiration, headaches (including migraines), rapid pulse, heart palpitations, bad breath, excessive vaginal discharge, hypoglycaemia.

This is quite a long list, and many of these symptoms can be caused by other conditions. However, if you suffer with at least four of these symptoms, there is a high probability that you have an allergy or sensitivity to a food you're eating.

How to identify a food sensitivity

Both of the eating plans in chapter six of this book exclude the foods most likely to cause a sensitivity. However, it's possible that a food you're eating is making you sick. If you do not experience significant health improvements after following the recommendations in this book for three months, it's possible you have a hidden food sensitivity.

There are several labs in that perform IgG tests to check for food intolerance. These tests can be very expensive, and the results are often not reliable.

A more reliable (and free) way of identifying problem foods is to remove the most common culprits from your diet for six weeks, and then assess your symptoms. When you reintroduce a food allergen back into your diet, eat it at least two to three times a day for three days to see if you notice an adverse reaction. If you do, stay away from the food for three months. After that time, you may be able to eat it safely as long as you don't go overboard; i.e. don't eat it every day of the week.

Foods that you might have a sensitivity to:

- Nuts
- Nightshade vegetables (tomatoes, eggplant, bell pepper, potatoes)
- Citrus fruits
- Yeast
- Vinegar

Chapter Four

The role of the gut and liver in autoimmune disease

Leaky gut syndrome

As you can see if you've read chapter three, there are many different contributors to the development of autoimmune disease. Apart from genetics, the second biggest factor determining whether you'll develop autoimmune disease or not is leaky gut syndrome. The more technical name for this condition is increased intestinal permeability, and it means just that; the intestinal lining has become more permeable than it should be. This is a problem because it allows wastes and toxins inside the intestines to get into your bloodstream, while also impairing the proper absorption of nutrients into your bloodstream.

Professor Alessio Fasano is a pediatric gastroenterologist and a world leader in research on leaky gut and its relationship to autoimmune disease. According to Professor Fasano, a leaky gut is necessary but not sufficient to develop an autoimmune disease.

That means you can't get an autoimmune disease unless you have a leaky gut

Chances are, if you're reading this book you have an autoimmune disease. That means your gut needs healing, so we strongly suggest you read this chapter carefully, as it's entirely relevant to your healing.

In a paper titled "Leaky gut and autoimmune diseases", Professor Fasano made the following statement: "In addition to genetic predisposition and exposure to triggering non-self antigens, the loss of the protective function of mucosal barriers that interact with the environment is necessary for autoimmunity to develop."[25]

What exactly is a leaky gut?

The lining of your intestines provides a very important barrier between your body and the outside world. The lining of your digestive tract is very much like the skin on the outside of your body; both of them protect your body against invasion by toxins or harmful organisms. The big difference is, the lining of your digestive tract is much thinner and more delicate.

Anything that's inside your gut isn't actually inside your body yet. If you accidentally swallow a marble it will travel from one end of your digestive system to the other end and leave your body. For anything to actually enter your body, it must get absorbed across your gastrointestinal lining. Once it has passed this barrier, it will truly be inside your body.

Leaky gut syndrome occurs when too much of the bad stuff gets in, while at the same time nutrient absorption is impaired

Structure of the small intestine

One of the main functions of your intestinal lining is to sort the good from the bad; to allow beneficial nutrients to enter your body, and prevent harmful substances from getting inside. Your mouth is the major entry point of foreign material into your body, so your gut has quite a lot of work to do. Approximately 70 to 80 percent of your body's immune cells lie within the lining of your small intestine, which makes sense because the gut is such an important interface between you and the outside world. This fact also explains why we place such a large emphasis on healing the gut, when trying to overcome any autoimmune disease.

Amazingly, your gut lining is comprised of a single layer of epithelial cells. These cells are called enterocytes and this single layer of cells is what you've got protecting your bloodstream from wastes and harmful substances. Immediately across this barrier you've got immune cells and a large network of blood vessels and lymphatic vessels, which carry absorbed nutrients to the tissues of your body.

The surface of the small intestine contains small, finger-like projections that protrude from the lining of the intestinal wall. These are called villi. Each villus is composed of many microvilli, and together, these structures form what is known as the brush border of the small intestine. See the diagram below. If you have been diagnosed with celiac disease, you'll know that the disease damages (flattens) the villi, and this is how celiac disease can create severe nutrient deficiencies.

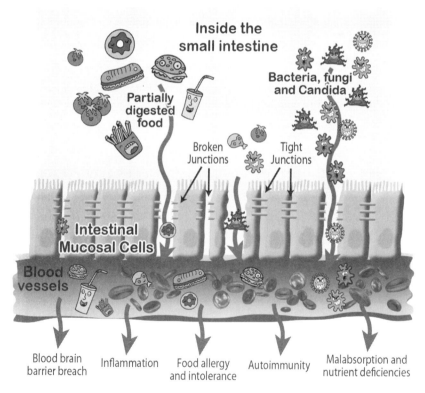

What does a leaky gut look like?

The purpose of villi is to increase the surface area of the intestinal walls. Increased surface area means increased space and facility for nutrient absorption. Your small intestine is designed in such a way as to enable you to absorb the greatest quantity of nutrients from your food as possible. Unfortunately your small intestine is very delicate, and several things can compromise its health, as you'll soon see.

Mechanism behind leaky gut

If you have a leaky gut, either the cells lining your small intestine (enterocytes), or the spaces between them get damaged sufficiently to create tiny microscopic holes in your gut lining. These holes are too small to be seen on examinations such as endoscopy or colonscopy. The holes allow the contents of your gut to leak into your bloodstream or lymphatic system. They first encounter the immune cells living within your gut lining, then make their way to your liver. When the liver becomes over burdened with toxins, they will spill out into your bloodstream and travel right throughout your body, entering every organ and tissue.

So what are these toxins that slip through a leaky gut? Incompletely digested food, bacteria, fungi, parasites, other microbes, heavy metals and wastes that your body is trying to excrete. If your gut is leaky you will also absorb bacterial toxins (endotoxins); these are highly damaging compounds that some bacteria secrete. Many people with a leaky gut have an excess of Candida in their gut, and Candida also secretes toxins that can make their way into your bloodstream and cause a variety of symptoms such as foggy head and mood disorders. Absorbing incompletely digested foods into your bloodstream is a sure fire way to develop food sensitivities. That's why people who have had a leaky gut for some time usually have several food allergies or intolerances, even if they don't know it.

If you have a leaky gut, it essentially means that the kind of wastes that make up your faeces are entering your bloodstream. A healthy small intestine should prevent that from happening; you are definitely not meant to have poo in your bloodstream. No wonder having a leaky gut can make you feel so terrible.

You can read the full list of symptoms of leaky gut syndrome on the following pages. You probably know that in all autoimmune diseases there is an excess of inflammation in the body. Far and away, the majority of this inflammation comes from the intestines if they are leaky, and if there are too many harmful microbes present inside.

A great deal of research has shown that the development of a leaky gut precedes the development of an autoimmune disease, and the flare up of an autoimmune disease that is in remission. In fact, a leaky gut has been found to be present in every autoimmune disease studied.

How exactly does the gut become leaky?

The cells making up your gut lining are held together by what are known as tight junctions, or gap junctions. These are proteins that extend outwards from the cells and join up with the neighbouring cell. The tight junctions open up when necessary, in order to allow beneficial nutrients to enter your bloodstream, but most of the time they remain tightly closed. Well, that's what's supposed to happen, but people with a leaky gut have tight junctions that remain open for too long.

If tight junctions remain open for too long, wastes from the intestines can seep into the body. It can also trigger death of the intestinal cell (called apoptosis). The most well known mechanism controlling the opening of gap junctions is via a compound called zonulin. Zonulin is a protein made by the enterocytes (intestinal cells), designed to regulate the opening and closing of gap junctions.

It has recently been discovered that many people with autoimmune disease manufacture too much zonulin, which keeps the gap junctions open for too long. The most studied disease related to zonulin is celiac disease. It has been shown that consumption of gluten by celiacs triggers oversecretion of zonulin. The same phenomenon has been well researched in people with type 1 diabetes. Excess zonulin production is being seen in an increasing number of autoimmune diseases and researchers are currently working on drugs that block zonulin release, in an attempt to prevent autoimmune disease by preventing the development of leaky gut. Gluten is a trigger for zonulin release even in individuals that don't have celiac disease.

How to know if you have a leaky gut

As mentioned, according to leading leaky gut researcher Professor Alessio Fasano, a leaky gut is necessary but not sufficient to cause an autoimmune disease. That means, if you've been diagnosed with an autoimmune disease, in all likelihood you have a leaky gut. Interestingly studies have shown increased intestinal permeability is also present in various other inflammatory conditions that are not autoimmune, including eczema, asthma, hay fever and autism. Individuals with those conditions are thought to be at increased risk of autoimmune disease some time in the future.

The following symptoms and conditions are common manifestations of leaky gut syndrome:

- Fatigue
- Joint pain
- Skin problems - eg. eczema, dermatitis, hives, skin rashes or itchy skin (remember that your skin on the outside is a reflection of what's happening to your skin on the inside [i.e. intestinal lining)
- Food sensitivities
- Autoimmune disease
- Cognitive problems - foggy head, poor memory, low motivation
- Respiratory problems - asthma, shortness of breath

- Anxiety
- Depression
- Muscle aches and pains and fibromyalgia
- Poor quality sleep and unrefreshing sleep
- Adrenal gland exhaustion
- Irritable bowel syndrome (IBS)
- Liver problems - raised liver enzymes, fatty liver disease, ache in the liver region (right upper portion of abdomen)
- Nutritional deficiencies - particularly iron, magnesium, vitamin B12 and vitamin D
- Inability to gain weight or lose weight

Those of you with autoimmune disease are probably quite familiar with several of these symptoms. Obviously, all those symptoms can have several different causes, but research has found a strong association between them and leaky gut.

It is important to realise that you don't need to experience any digestive symptoms in order to have a leaky gut. You can't feel whether your gut is leaky or not. It is easy to imagine someone with Crohn's disease or ulcerative colitis suffering with a leaky gut, with the dreadful abdominal cramps, diarrhea and mucus in the stool that these people experience. However, the development of leaky gut syndrome precedes these diseases. Leaky gut came first; long before the diarrhea or abdominal cramps started. Some people with celiac disease don't experience any digestive discomfort at all, despite having severe damage to their intestines, as seen on a biopsy.

Even if you have a cast iron stomach and rarely ever get an upset gut, chances are you have a leaky gut if you've been diagnosed with an autoimmune disease or inflammatory disease. So please don't think this chapter of the book isn't relevant to you if you don't experience any digestive symptoms.

Is there a test for leaky gut?

There is a test called the lactulose-mannitol test, which can assess your degree of intestinal permeability. The test involves drinking a small amount of lactulose and mannitol and then having your urine collected for the next five to six hours. Lactulose and mannitol are both types of sugar, but only mannitol is small enough to get absorbed through the intestinal lining and end up in the bloodstream, in healthy individuals. Lactulose is a larger molecule that can't get absorbed through the gut, although people with a leaky gut will absorb it into their bloodstream. Once in your bloodstream, your kidneys will excrete it into your urine in several hours. The leakier your gut, the more lactulose will be present in your urine.

Do we recommend you have this test? Not really; at least not initially. As we've said, if you're reading this book, there's a very high probability you have a leaky gut. Even if you don't, by following our recommendations for healing leaky gut, you should experience great improvements in your autoimmune condition and your overall wellbeing. You will be able to know whether your gut permeability has improved or not based on how you feel and whether your health improves.

What causes a leaky gut?

The short answer is very many things.

It could be said that living in modern society is enough to give you a leaky gut. The list below may look overwhelming and make you feel like there's no hope in improving your gut health but please be assured, this is not the case. There are degrees of leaky gut, and you can achieve a great improvement that's sufficient enough to heal your autoimmune disease and enable you to feel well.

The following factors all increase intestinal permeability:

- Alcohol.
- Non-Steroidal Anti-inflammatory drugs eg. aspirin, naproxen, ibuprofen, meloxicam.
- Dysbiosis (imbalance between good and bad microbes in the gut).
- Candida infection.
- Small intestinal bacterial overgrowth (SIBO).
- Inefficient digestion resulting from deficiencies of stomach acid, bile or digestive enzymes.
- Gastrointestinal infections i.e. parasites, food poisoning or gastroenteritis.
- Intense or chronic stress.
- A high sugar or refined carbohydrate diet.
- Gluten.
- Intense exercise, such as marathon running temporarily causes increased intestinal permeability.
- Food allergy or intolerance.
- Lectins, saponins and alkaloids found in some foods such as grains and legumes.
- Nutritional deficiencies, particularly zinc and vitamin A.
- The oral contraceptive pill.

That's quite a long list, but fortunately there are effective strategies that can heal your gut.

How is leaky gut linked to autoimmune disease?

The leading theory to explain the connection between leaky gut and autoimmune disease is called molecular mimicry. When wastes and toxins in your gut are allowed entry into your bloodstream, your immune system naturally becomes alarmed and starts attacking these unwanted substances with antibodies and inflammatory chemicals.

If this is allowed to continue for years, your immune system can become overwhelmed and start confusing the cells of your own body with some of the harmful substances leaking through your gut. Studies have shown that the surface protein molecules of some intestinal microbes closely resemble some of the cells of your own body, such as your thyroid gland, your joints, your pancreas and other tissues. If your immune cells have been making antibodies against those microbes leaking through your gut for a long time, eventually they can start forming antibodies against your own body. Thus you have the beginning of an autoimmune disease.

Having a leaky gut also places an enormous strain on your liver, because all blood from your intestines heads straight for your liver first (via the hepatic portal vein). If you are suffering with dysbiosis and your gut is excessively permeable, a great deal of metabolic wastes and bacterial toxins (endotoxins) will arrive at your liver each day. The liver can become chronically inflamed and spew inflammatory chemicals into your bloodstream. The chronic overstimulation of your immune system that results also raises the risk of autoimmune disease. An overburdened liver will not be able to cleanse and filter your bloodstream well, and therefore your immune system will suffer.

How to fix a leaky gut

Healing a leaky gut is the number one priority in order to overcome autoimmune disease. Stopping the excessive influx of toxins into your bloodstream will take the stress off your immune system and liver. This will greatly reduce the inflammatory chemicals in your bloodstream.

Healing a leaky gut will also improve your ability to absorb nutrients. That means you'll obtain more nourishment from the food you eat and supplements you take. People with autoimmune disease have typically been deficient in several vitamins and minerals for a long time. This weakens the immune system and increases the risk of infections and other health problems. It is always a pleasure to see a patient's health thrive once their gut health is restored.

Healing a leaky gut involves 4 components:

1. Remove foods that irritate the gut and encourage increased intestinal permeability.

2. Correct dysbiosis and/or small intestinal bacterial overgrowth. This means, restore the balance of good and bad gut microbes, in the correct location.

3. Improve digestive function.

4. Heal and seal the intestinal lining with specific foods and nutrients.

We will now explain each component in more detail.

1. Remove foods that irritate the gut

The worst offenders are gluten, dairy products, legumes and sugar. Other potentially problematic foods include all grains, eggs, nightshade vegetables (tomatoes, potatoes, bell peppers and eggplant) and nuts. In addition, any food to which you have an allergy or intolerance can inflame your gut when you consume it.

2. Correct dysbiosis and/or Small Intestinal Bacterial Overgrowth (SIBO)

Dysbiosis means having too much bad bacteria, Candida or other microbes in the bowel and not enough good microbes. Another common problem is Small Intestinal Bacterial Overgrowth (SIBO). This means there are too many microbes growing in the small intestine, where they shouldn't be. They aren't necessarily bad bugs, they're just living in the wrong place. Dysbiosis and SIBO cause leaky gut syndrome and nutrient deficiencies. They are covered in detail later in this chapter.

3. **Improve digestive function**

Deficiencies of stomach acid, bile and digestive enzymes are very common in people with a leaky gut. It is critically important that you digest your food as thoroughly as possible. This will enable you to absorb the maximum amount of nutrients from your food, but there's also another reason. If you don't digest your food properly, it will literally rot or ferment inside your gut. The residues of undigested carbohydrate in particular, will act as food for harmful gut microbes, or encourage their growth in the small intestine, creating SIBO and leaky gut.

4. **Heal and seal the gut**

There are specific foods and nutrients that help to reduce inflammation in the digestive tract and restore the health of the intestinal lining. We need to make it a stronger barrier, so that you don't keep absorbing toxins and wastes into your bloodstream.

The most important substances to heal a leaky gut are glutamine, bone broth, berberine, zinc and vitamin A. They are discussed in more detail in chapter seven.

Dysbiosis and Small Intestinal Bacterial Overgrowth (SIBO)

The human gastrointestinal tract contains 10^{14} microorganisms. This is approximately ten times the number of cells that make up the entire human body. So microbes outnumber your own body's cells by ten to one. There are more than 1000 different species of microbes that call your body their home, and the microbes in your gut weigh over 3 pounds! [26] It's a staggering thought, and it highlights just how important your gut is to your overall health. It seems humans are really just a life support system for bugs!

Different species of bacteria prefer living in different areas, so the bacteria in your small intestine is different to the bacteria in your large intestine. Well, that's what's supposed to happen, but things can go wrong and this is typical in patients with autoimmune disease.

The collection of bugs living in your digestive tract is collectively known as your gut microbiome. Because these bugs are beneficial to your health, they're known as probiotics. It's not just bacteria that live inside your digestive tract; you'll also find yeast, viruses and archaea (similar organisms to bacteria).

What functions does your gut microbiome perform for you?

The microbes in your gut are there for very important reasons. You would not survive without them. The number of biochemical reactions they perform rival those of your liver. Clearly, you want your gut bugs to be as healthy as possible. Taking a probiotic supplement or eating fermented foods will give you the benefits listed below.

So far, researchers have determined that your gut microbiome performs the following functions:

- Regulation of immune system function. Your gut bugs help to protect you from infections by inhibiting the binding of pathogenic bacteria to your intestinal cells. They regulate IgA production in the gut and help to prevent allergic reactions. They also help to maintain immune tolerance by improving the health of T-regulatory cells. This means your gut bugs are supposed to help you recognise your own cells and organs, and make sure you don't attack them. This function goes horribly wrong in people with autoimmune disease. A healthy gut microbiome helps to balance the different arms of the immune system. Specifically it helps to balance Th1, Th2 and Th3 immune cells. An imbalance between these different cell types is a feature of all autoimmune diseases.

- Maintenance of normal gut motility. Healthy gut bugs help to normalise bowel function, so that you don't suffer from constipation or diarrhea. They also help to maintain more subtle gut movements called cleansing waves, which help to prevent a build up of microbes in the small intestine.

- Production of short chain fatty acids, including butyric acid, propionic acid and acetic acid. These fatty acids provide nourishment for the cells lining your intestines and they help to reduce the risk of bowel cancer. These short chain fatty acids also help your body to absorb minerals, including zinc, iron, magnesium, copper and calcium.

- Maintenance of a healthy mood. Alterations in the gut flora can increase the risk of depression and anxiety. Research in this area is increasing at a rapid rate.

- Weight maintenance. There is a strong relationship between the types of bugs in your gut and your body weight. Having too many harmful microbes leads to the increased production of inflammatory chemicals. These inflammatory chemicals can create insulin resistance (syndrome X) and also place enormous stress on the liver, impairing its fat burning and detoxification abilities.

- Assistance with digestion. Your gut bugs contain enzymes that help you digest your food more thoroughly. They particularly help with the digestion of starch and fiber; helping you to extract more nutrients from plant foods. Gut microflora help to break down phytic acid in foods like nuts and seeds, improving the digestibility of minerals in these foods.

- Synthesis of vitamins, particularly B vitamins and vitamin K2.

- Enhancement of the absorption of fatty acids and fat soluble nutrients such as vitamins A, D, K and E. Deficiencies of these nutrients is very common in people with autoimmune disease.

- Protection from infection by directing the production of antibodies against invading pathogens.

In short, your microbiome plays a critical role in the maintenance of a healthy immune system. It helps to prevent excessively high levels of inflammation in your body. Excessive inflammation is a feature of all autoimmune disease, therefore improving the health of your microbiome is critical. Achieving a healthy microbiome involves having a healthy population of gut microbes living in the correct numbers, in the correct location and in appropriate diversity. Unfortunately, a lot of things can go wrong, and this ideal is often not present.

Healthy gut bugs can help to keep you thin

Your body weight is determined by a large number of different factors. Researchers have come to realise that the "calories in, calories out" theory of weight loss is far too simplistic and doesn't take each individual's metabolism into account. A range of different hormones, along with the health of your thyroid gland, your liver, your adrenal glands and other organs all help to determine your body weight.

Interestingly, your microbiome also plays a hand in determining your weight. Research conducted on mice gave us some very interesting clues. When the gut bacteria from lean mice is transplanted into the guts of obese mice, those mice soon become lean. The reverse is also true; thin mice can become obese if implanted with the gut bugs from obese mice. The mice that became obese also developed insulin resistance (also called syndrome X, metabolic syndrome and pre-diabetes).

Subsequent studies have shown that obese people (and animals) tend to have plenty of bacteria from the Firmicutes family, which includes Lactobacillus bacteria, which is found in yogurt and most probiotic supplements. This family of bacteria is very beneficial, and required for good health for numerous reasons.

Thin people tend to also have a lot of bacteria from the Bacteroidetes family in their gut. You can't buy Bacteroidetes bacteria in supplement form, but you can eat the foods they require in order to flourish. These foods are polyphenols. Polyphenols are antioxidants abundantly found in brightly coloured fruits and vegetables. They also happen to be prebiotics for Bacteroidetes. Apart from brightly coloured foods like berries, other excellent sources of polyphenols include green tea, coffee, chocolate and extra virgin olive oil. Coffee and chocolate may not be appropriate for everyone reading this book, but good quality 90 percent cocoa dark chocolate is an extremely healthy food that anyone would benefit from. This type of chocolate is usually dairy free and the sugar content is so low that it's negligible.

What is dysbiosis?

This is a general term used to describe harmful alterations in the quantity or quality of gut microbes. It is essentially an imbalance between beneficial and harmful microorganisms living in your digestive system. This situation can have a profoundly negative effect on your digestive function, on the lining of your intestines (promoting leaky gut syndrome) and, ultimately, on your immune health. High levels of gut dysbiosis create high levels of inflammation in your body.

Small Intestinal Bacterial Overgrowth (SIBO)

This is the most common type of dysbiosis and emerging research has shown it is a significant factor in the development of most types of autoimmune diseases. The biggest reason why SIBO is so harmful is because it creates leaky gut syndrome.

SIBO is defined as an increased number and/or abnormal types of bacteria in the small intestine

The condition encompasses yeast overgrowth such as Candida too, but excess bacteria is more common and a bigger problem. There is not supposed to be a lot of bacteria in your small intestine. This part of your intestine is designed for nutrient digestion and absorption. Most of the bugs in your gut are supposed to live in your colon (large intestine). How does the bacteria end up in your small intestine? It can either travel upwards from your colon, or downwards from your mouth. The far more common scenario is where the bugs travel up from your large intestine.

The bacteria present in SIBO are not necessarily bad bacteria, like the ones that cause gastroenteritis or food poisoning. The problem is, the bacteria are just in the wrong place.

The fiber in fruits, vegetables, nuts and other plant foods is not digestible by us, but it is digestible by gut bacteria. Your gut bugs break down fiber and starch and use it as their food supply. This is a good thing if it happens in the colon. The break down of fiber and starch (called fermentation) in the small intestine creates gases and toxins. This can make you feel bloated and it can cause symptoms of irritable bowel syndrome such as abdominal cramps, gas, diarrhea or constipation. New research has shown that many cases of irritable bowel syndrome are actually caused by SIBO.

There are other problems with fermentation happening in your small intestine. Fermentation is what occurs when bacteria eat. Along with gases, bacteria and yeast also produce several toxins while they are feeding on the fibers and starches you've eaten. In fact, any food you were not able to digest thoroughly can become food for bacteria and yeast and encourage an overgrowth of these microbes. That's why good digestion is so critical for anyone with autoimmune disease and anyone who wants to overcome a leaky gut.

The lining of your small intestine is very thin; you may remember that it's only one cell thick. The excess bacteria in the small intestine of someone living with SIBO cause inflammatory damage to the lining of the small intestine. The damaged, leaky gut now absorbs those toxins, plus other wastes. They get into your bloodstream and travel straight to your liver. It's not surprising then to learn that SIBO is a strong contributing factor to liver inflammation and fatty liver. This is covered in more detail later in this chapter.

Symptoms of Small Intestinal Bacterial Overgrowth (SIBO)

The symptoms of SIBO can vary enormously from person to person. Some people get terrible IBS (irritable bowel syndrome) symptoms such as bloating, flatulence, burping, abdominal pains, constipation or diarrhea. Other people get no digestive symptoms at all; they just experience some of the harmful consequences of SIBO, listed below.

The research on SIBO is still in its infancy, but there are several well established conditions that may result from an overgrowth of bacteria in the small intestine. These include the following:

- Nutrient deficiencies, particularly iron deficiency. SIBO can result in iron deficiency because the lining of the intestines becomes inflamed and this impairs nutrient absorption. Iron deficiency can also occur because the bacteria steal iron from your food and use it for their own metabolism. Deficiencies in B vitamins and vitamin D are also common.

- Muscle cramps, spasms or restless legs syndrome. Muscle cramps and spasms are usually caused by magnesium deficiency due to malabsorption. Iron deficiency is strongly correlated with restless legs syndrome as well. Many people need to supplement with both iron and magnesium to resolve this condition (as well as healing their gut of course). The best test to check if you're iron deficient is a blood test for ferritin.

- Joint pain.

- Fibromyalgia.

- Fatigue.

- Multiple food sensitivities.

- Inflammation of the liver (raised liver enzymes).

- Skin problems, including eczema, acne rosacea, rashes or itchy skin.

- Refractory celiac disease (celiac disease that doesn't resolve on a gluten free diet).

- Strong sugar or carbohydrate cravings. The excess bacteria and yeast in the small intestine want to be fed. They need carbohydrate in order to survive, so you're likely to have big cravings for these foods.

Causes of Small Intestinal Bacterial Overgrowth (SIBO)

Your body has a number of protective mechanisms to guard against the development of SIBO. The condition develops when too many of these mechanisms aren't working.

The following conditions all increase the risk of SIBO:

- Insufficient stomach acid. Your stomach is supposed to be very acidic. Strong acid is a good disinfectant and helps to kill bacteria and prevent too much of it from travelling down into your small intestine. Stomach acid also activates digestive enzymes, which enable you to digest your food properly. Insufficient stomach acid is a very common problem in those with autoimmune disease. It's also one of the biggest causes of food allergies.

- Bile from the gallbladder and pancreatic digestive juices also help to prevent excessive bacterial growth in the small intestine if they are produced in sufficient quantities. Often they are not. People with pancreatitis usually have SIBO. Excessive bacteria in the small intestine can travel to the pancreas and inflame it, raising the risk of pancreatitis.

- Abnormal anatomy of the small intestine. A number of conditions can raise the risk of SIBO, including bowel adhesions after surgery, bowel strictures (narrowing of the intestines) associated with Crohn's disease; endometriosis that has created lesions on the bowel; weight loss surgery including gastric bypass and gastric sleeve.

- Abnormal function of the ileocaecal valve. This is a valve that separates the large intestine from the small intestine. It is designed to prevent the upwards movement of the contents of the large intestine into the small intestine. Over eating to the point of discomfort and bloating in the large intestine can inhibit the proper function of this valve. This can allow bacteria from the colon to travel into the small intestine and promote the development of SIBO.

- Abnormalities in intestinal motility. Your intestinal tract is not just a tube through which food travels. Your intestines actually do quite a bit of work to help push everything through at the correct pace. You may have heard of peristalsis; this is the name given to the intestinal contractions that move food through your digestive tract. There is another type of far more subtle motility called cleansing waves, or migrating motor complex.

The cleansing waves start in your stomach and they gently sweep undigested food particles, bacteria and other debris from your stomach, through your small intestine and into your large intestine for eventual removal from your body. These cleansing waves are designed to keep your stomach and small intestine relatively free of bacteria compared to your colon. The cleansing waves are activated by cells in your small intestine approximately every 90 minutes, but only occur when your body isn't digesting food. Therefore, they predominantly occur during the night, and also several hours after a meal, provided you haven't had a snack.

You are supposed to have approximately nine cleansing waves per day, but studies have shown that some people with SIBO have 70 percent less cleansing waves than they're supposed to

This makes it much easier for high numbers of bacteria to take up residence in your small intestine, where they shouldn't be. Eating between meals or grazing throughout the day reduces the number of cleansing waves you'll have. That's one of the reasons we recommend you try not to snack. It is best to have three meals a day and let your digestive system rest and cleanse itself between meals. Digesting food is hard work for your body and it takes away from the energy required to heal your immune system. Medication that can cause constipation, such as opiod pain relievers and some antidepressants can also reduce the number of cleansing waves.

Some gut infections can inhibit cleansing waves. This is because some pathogens that are responsible for causing food poisoning or gastroenteritis release toxins that inhibit the function of the migrating motor complex. This means it becomes harder for your body to excrete the pathogenic bug responsible for the infection. Life really is a battle for survival and the harmful pathogens want to stay in your gut longer and try to prevent you from flushing them out.

In some cases following an intestinal infection, an autoimmune reaction can occur to the cells of your intestine that control the cleansing waves[27]. This is one explanation for how gastroenteritis or food poisoning can be a trigger for the development of SIBO and a subsequent autoimmune disease. The good news is that beneficial probiotics help to promote regular cleansing waves. That's how probiotic supplements and fermented foods can help to prevent SIBO.

- Insufficient intestinal secretion of immunoglobulin A (secretory IgA). This is a type of antiseptic paint secreted by the intestinal cells that helps to keep levels of bacteria in check. Deficiencies of IgA are common in patients with autoimmune disease. There is a blood test that can check for this. Probiotics help to increase IgA secretion.

- Use of stomach acid blocking medication, particularly proton pump inhibitors. These are some of the most commonly prescribed drugs in the world and examples include Nexium, Losec, Zoton and Pariet. They are prescribed for reflux, heartburn and peptic ulcers. It is very rare for any of those conditions to actually be caused by excessive stomach acid. The real causes include SIBO and food intolerance. However, these drugs usually do offer some symptom relief, so they are routinely prescribed. Blocking stomach acid means you lose its disinfectant properties and some research showed that at least 50 percent of people taking a proton pump inhibitor develop SIBO[28].

- Diabetic neuropathy is a risk factor for SIBO because when the nerves get damaged by excessively high blood sugar this impairs normal intestinal contractions.

- In elderly individuals there's a strong prevalence of SIBO at 75 years of age and greater.

- Diverticulitis significantly increases the risk of SIBO. This makes sense because the bowel pockets typically become infected with bacteria. In fact, they act like breeding grounds for harmful bugs, where they cannot be flushed out of the bowel in regular bowel motions.

- There is a very high incidence of SIBO in people with celiac disease. This is usually because celiacs tend to produce insufficient stomach acid and digestive enzymes.

- Fructose intolerance, FODMAP problems and IBS (irritable bowel syndrome) often go hand in hand with SIBO. FODMAPs are fermentable fibers found in many different foods, including fruit and vegetables. This topic is covered in more detail in chapter six. Not being able to digest fructose or fermentable fibers properly will leave lots of food for bacteria and yeast to feast on in the small intestine. Therefore, having an intolerance to these foods usually indicates you have SIBO. Correcting the balance of microbes in your intestines, and increasing digestive enzymes improves the ability to digest fructose and FODMAPs in most cases.

If you think you may have SIBO, we strongly recommend you follow the stage 2 eating plan in chapter six. It has been specifically designed to help eradicate excess bacteria and yeast in the small intestine.

Testing for SIBO

How can you find out for sure whether or not you have SIBO? There are various tests, but none of them are perfect. The gold standard test involves aspirating (sucking up) some fluid from the small intestine via enteroscopy. That means you'd be sedated while a long tube with a tiny camera and a syringe on the end of it are passed through your mouth, all the way down into your small intestine. The fluid that's obtained then gets cultured and analysed for the types and numbers of bacterial strains. It's not a pleasant test and it's not that reliable because some strains of bacteria can't be cultured well in laboratory settings; they tend to die as soon as they're removed from their home. Also, bacteria tend to form a biofilm on the intestinal wall, therefore not much of that can be obtained from intestinal fluid.

Breath testing for SIBO is a much more popular test. This involves testing the breath for levels of hydrogen and methane. Humans don't manufacture these gases, so if there's too much in your intestines, it can only come from bacterial fermentation of carbohydrates you're not digesting properly. In healthy people, hydrogen and methane producing bacteria live mostly in the large intestine, therefore the gases that are produced get expelled as flatus. In a person with SIBO, too much of this bacteria lives higher up in the small intestine, therefore the gases can be measured via a breath test.

There is controversy over which testing method is best - glucose or lactulose. The breath test is not 100 percent reliable. Lactulose breath tests can be difficult to interpret, and glucose tests are good for detecting bacterial overgrowth in the first part of the small intestine, but not so good at detecting bacteria further down towards the large intestine.

For this test, you would be given a sugary solution to drink that contains either glucose or lactulose. You'll then be asked to blow into a bag every 15 or 30 minutes, over the course of 1.5 to three hours.

Another problem with the breath test is it is good at detecting overgrowth of bacteria that feed on fructose, lactose and sorbitol, but not good at detecting bugs that feed off fructans, mannitol and galactans. These are various fermentable fibers known by the acronym FODMAPs.

SIBO breath tests usually cost around $100. There are various labs in the United States that perform them, see www.sibotest.com for more information. Because these tests are not terribly accurate, we recommend you follow the stage 2 protocol in chapter six if you suspect you have SIBO. This eating plan is a low FODMAP diet, which excludes highly fermentable fibers from your diet. You will probably notice an improvement in your digestive health on this diet. If it does not resolve your symptoms, you may consider getting a breath test.

Other clues you may have SIBO

If you're uncertain about whether to get a breath test for SIBO or not, there are other clues that indicate you probably have SIBO. If you have irritable bowel syndrome and feel better after a course of antibiotics, you probably have SIBO. This is because antibiotics can kill off some of the excess bacteria in your intestines. Therefore, some people experience symptom relief for a few weeks, but after that, the bacteria usually grows back unless the underlying cause is addressed.

Another clue is feeling better after a bout of diarrhea. This does not apply to people who regularly experience diarrhea as a feature of their autoimmune disease (e.g. Crohn's disease or ulcerative colitis). In people with SIBO, getting a one off bout of diarrhea can leave them feeling significantly better in terms of energy level and overall health because the diarrhea flushes out some of the bacterial overgrowth.

Another clue that you may have SIBO is generally feeling bloated from eating any type of carbohydrate rich food, and even getting bloated after eating a large serving of vegetables such as broccoli, onion or cabbage.

How to overcome SIBO

As mentioned, there are a lot of negative health consequences from having small intestinal bacterial overgrowth. In people with autoimmune disease, it can be one of the biggest triggers of the disease and it can stand in the way of your efforts to repair a leaky gut and heal your intestines.

The conventional treatment of SIBO involves the use of antibiotics. The most commonly used antibiotics include rifaximin (brand name Xifaxan), vancomycin (brand name Vancocin), metronidazole (brand name Flagyl) and neomycin (brand name Neosulf). Neomycin is usually only added to the mix in people who suffer with constipation, because it's good for stimulating intestinal contractions.

All of these antibiotics mostly stay in the intestines. They are not absorbed into the bloodstream in significant quantities. The good thing about that is the antibiotics are less likely to reduce levels of beneficial microbes in other parts of the body such as the urinary tract, genital region and respiratory tract. Therefore they're less likely to create side effects like thrush.

We do not recommend you use antibiotics to overcome SIBO. Antibiotics can have harmful side effects, particularly to the liver and kidneys

They can also wipe out too much of the good bacteria in your gut, leaving you more prone to infections by pathogenic bacteria. The other problem with antibiotic treatment of SIBO is the benefits are only short lived. In the vast majority of cases the treatment is only effective for several weeks to months. One study showed that successful antibiotic treatment of SIBO only lasted for 22 days! [29] To get around this, some doctors are recommending continuous antibiotic use for their patients. This is definitely not what we'd recommend. If you want to permanently eradicate SIBO, you need to address all the reasons it developed in the first place.

Natural remedies for overcoming SIBO

An interesting article was published in the medical journal Global Advances in Health and Medicine called Herbal Therapy is Equivalent to Rifaximin for Small Intestinal Bacterial Overgrowth. The conclusion to the study read: "Herbal therapies are at least as effective as rifaximin for resolution of SIBO by lactulose breath testing. Herbals also appear to be as effective as triple antibiotic therapy for SIBO rescue therapy for rifaximin non-responders. Further, prospective studies are needed to validate these findings and explore additional alternative therapies in patients with refractory SIBO." [30]

We agree with that outcome. Herbal remedies are much safer and just as effective as antibiotics in the eradication of SIBO.

The most beneficial herbs include:

- oregano oil
- clove oil
- berberine
- peppermint oil
- garlic
- thyme oil
- coconut oil

You can find these herbs and essential oils in supplement form. Essential oils work best when they are in enteric coated capsules, so they don't dissolve until they get to your small intestine.

Diet for SIBO eradication

Changing your diet is critical if you want to overcome SIBO for good. The aim here is to starve the bacteria and yeast of their food supply so they can die off. Some physicians recommend an elemental diet for the treatment of SIBO. Elemental diets are liquid preparations of predigested food. They are often used in hospitals to feed patients who are unconscious or not able to eat regular foods. They are a bit like meal replacements but all the nutrients have been broken down into their building blocks so they don't require any work to digest. This also means the nutrients are digested rapidly, so they aren't given a chance to feed bacteria in the small intestine; therefore the bacteria die.

There are lots of problems with elemental diets though:

- The preparations are expensive
- They generally taste terrible
- They contain dodgy ingredients like high fructose corn syrup, vegetable oil and genetically modified ingredients
- They are generally only recommended to be used for two to four weeks and it takes longer than that to eradicate SIBO.

Elemental diets can sometimes be necessary or even lifesaving, particularly in people with Crohn's disease or ulcerative colitis, where the intestines are extremely inflamed and damaged.

Fortunately, in the vast majority of cases, SIBO can be corrected with a low FODMAP, low starch diet and herbal antimicrobials

The stage 2 eating plan in chapter six is specifically designed to eradicate SIBO. You will get better results if you take a course of herbal antimicrobials for SIBO for a period of approximately six weeks before implementing the low FODMAP diet. Therefore, keep eating the fermentable starches while taking the herbs, and start the low FODMAP diet afterwards.

That means, if you have SIBO, follow the stage 1 eating plan in chapter six first for 6 weeks, while taking herbal antimicrobials to eradicate SIBO. After that time, move on to the stage 2 eating plan (low FODMAP diet).

You may have a yeast or fungal overgrowth

Sometimes yeast overgrowth is a bigger problem than bacterial overgrowth. This is a very common condition in people with immune system problems but conventional medicine doesn't have any safe and effective treatments.

Some types of fungal infections are well known. For example, AIDS patients usually get severe fungal overgrowth and they require long term treatment with powerful antifungal drugs. These drugs are very liver toxic, by the way. Diabetics are more prone to fungal infections because yeast loves sugar and requires it for its growth, and diabetics have high blood sugar. Women tend to get thrush after a course of antibiotics, and infants often suffer with fungal skin infections such as cradle cap.

These types of fungal infections are obvious because they can be seen, but fungal infections are sometimes much more subtle. This makes them very hard to identify and hard to treat. All yeast infections originate in the gut; from there they can spread to other parts of the body and create a variety of symptoms and health problems. The problem with suffering a yeast overgrowth in the gut is the fact that it creates a leaky gut and, as you know, that's the start of a whole lot of other problems. Also, the toxins released from the yeast travel throughout your bloodstream and chronically stress your immune system. This worsens the high levels of inflammation already present in the body of someone with autoimmune disease.

Typical symptoms that indicate you may be suffering from a yeast infection include:

- Fatigue
- Abdominal bloating
- Thrush or vaginal itching in women
- Anal itching

- Itchy ears (inside the ears)
- Frequent bladder infections or irritation of the bladder where no infection can be found
- Foggy head and inability to concentrate
- A history of frequent antibiotic use
- A history of oral contraceptive use
- A history of steroid use, such as for asthma or for an autoimmune disease
- Allergies
- Sensitivity to strong smells, particularly perfumes and laundry detergents
- Eczema
- Fungal nail infections
- Strong cravings for sugar and/or high carbohydrate foods

There aren't any reliable tests for checking for a subtle yeast infection. Blood tests and stool tests aren't very accurate because we all have some yeast in our bodies; it's only a problem if yeast grows in excessively high numbers. If you suffer with several of the symptoms in the list above, there's a good chance you have yeast overgrowth.

How to treat a yeast infection

If conventional medicine recognises a yeast infection, prescription antifungal drugs are usually recommended. Nystatin is a commonly used antifungal. The good thing about Nystatin is it doesn't have any harmful side effects because it remains in the gut. It is given in capsule form and the medication doesn't get absorbed into your bloodstream. Therefore, it can be good for killing off excessive yeast like Candida in the gastrointestinal tract. Unfortunately, many fungal organisms are resistant to Nystatin, so it's often not very effective at controlling yeast overgrowth.

There are stronger medications that have the ability to kill yeast. Some examples include Diflucan, Sporonox and Lamasil. Unfortunately, these drugs are very toxic to the liver. Anyone who takes them needs to have a blood test called a liver function test approximately every six weeks to make sure they are not damaging the liver. Some patients feel dramatically better after a course of one of these antifungal drugs, but we do not recommend them. There are far safer ways of helping your body to beat a yeast infection.

Natural ways of overcoming a yeast infection

Avoid consuming sugar, gluten, grains, dairy products and any foods to which you have a sensitivity. Following the stage 1 or 2 eating plans in chapter six would help you overcome a yeast infection.

There are several herbs and essential oils with natural antifungal properties; these include oregano oil, garlic, berberine, thyme oil, garlic and clove oil.

Coconut oil has antifungal properties and research has shown it is quite effective at killing Candida[31]. It is a type of beneficial fat called lauric acid, found in coconut oil that is antimicrobial and effective at killing several different pathogens. Coconut oil also has the ability to kill Helicobacter pylori, which is the bacteria that is linked with stomach ulcers and stomach cancer[32]. If you want good overall health, include some coconut oil in your diet each day. You can cook with it, add it to smoothies or just eat it straight off the spoon.

Make sure your home or workplace is not contaminated with mould. Dr Peter Dingle is a toxicologist who has written an excellent book on the subject called "Is your home making you sick?"

Saccharomyces boulardii is a type of beneficial, non-pathogenic yeast originally isolated from the surface of lichee nuts. It is widely used around the world to treat diarrhea, but is effective for a range of digestive problems. Treatment with Saccharomyces boulardii is commonly called "yeast against yeast", because it is a good yeast that is able to clear bad yeast (and bacteria) out of the gut. Clinical trials have shown the effectiveness of S. boulardii in the treatment and prevention of diarrhea caused by Clostridium difficile; antibiotic induced diarrhea and traveler's diarrhea[33, 34]. S. boulardii also has the ability to increase secretory IgA production in the gut[35]. Secretory IgA acts like an antiseptic paint; helping to protect the gut from infection and invasion. It also helps to maintain gut barrier function, and improves leaky gut.

Dealing with a die off reaction

Killing off yeast and harmful bacteria is a good thing, but you need to be aware that sometimes the dead microbes release enough byproducts to cause a "die off" reaction that could make you feel worse before you feel better. The "die off" symptoms may take up to a week to completely resolve. You can minimise the symptoms by getting as much rest and sleep as possible, and drinking lots of water, green tea or herbal tea.

It is also very helpful to take two to three activated charcoal capsules every four to six hours during the day. The charcoal will bind with the toxins produced by yeast or bacteria and carry them out of your body in bowel motions. This will reduce the amount of toxins that get absorbed into your bloodstream and stress your liver and immune system. Activated charcoal can also reduce your absorption of nutritional supplements or prescription medication, therefore it needs to be taken on an empty stomach; at least two hours before or after taking supplements or medication.

Taking a magnesium supplement at the same time can have a mild laxative effect, helping to remove the toxins with the charcoal more thoroughly from your body. Some people can get a bit constipated by charcoal, and magnesium helps to prevent that. You could take one teaspoon of Magnesium Ultra Potent powder twice daily.

Fix your digestion

You have probably heard the expression "You are what you eat". In fact, it's more accurate to say "You are what you absorb". Eating healthy food is vitally important if you want to heal an autoimmune disease, but digesting and absorbing that food well is even more vital. Poor digestion is extremely common among people with autoimmune disease. It is a major factor in why they developed an autoimmune disease in the first place.

Many people are concerned about environmental chemicals, pollutants in air and water; chemicals in personal care products, cleaning products and so on. They are all valid concerns and we urge you to minimise your exposure to environmental chemicals as much as possible. However, it's important to realise that the greatest source of toxicity in your body, are the toxins coming from a toxic gut. Your gut is toxic if you're not digesting your food properly and if you have an overgrowth of the wrong bugs in the wrong places.

Excess inflammation is a feature of every autoimmune disease. The inflammation can come from a variety of sources; the gut is one of the biggest. Some researchers have gone so far as to say "increased systemic inflammation is almost, if not always, a sign of dysbiosis and increased translocation of toxins of bacterial origin, such as endotoxin".[36]

That means the greatest source of inflammation is often a toxic gut

Endotoxins are toxins released by certain strains of gram negative bacteria in the gut. They are highly inflammatory and when they get into your bloodstream and travel to your liver, they can cause significant liver inflammation. They can make you feel absolutely dreadful, with symptoms such as exhaustion, nausea, foggy head, aches and pains, poor quality sleep, depression or anxiety.

Lipopolysaccharide is an example of an endotoxin and it's one of the most inflammatory substances in nature.

Clearly, you need to clean up your gut if you want to reduce inflammation in your body

Your gut is the primary interface between you and the outside world. Remember that your intestinal lining is made up of a single layer of epithelial cells. On the other side of that one layer of cells lies a teeming mass of bacteria, fungi, viruses, wastes and foreign proteins. The leakier your gut, the more of these toxins your immune system will have to deal with. This situation will be even worse if you have dysbiosis and if you're not digesting your food properly.

If you aren't breaking your food down into its simplest components and absorbing them well, you'll be leaving behind waste that becomes food for the bacteria and yeast inside your digestive tract. Inefficient digestion leaves food scraps behind, and bad bugs will have a party feasting on what you haven't been able to digest so you want your digestion to be as thorough as possible. Unfortunately, deficiency of stomach acid, digestive enzymes and bile is typical in patients with autoimmune disease. This situation must be corrected if you want to clean up your gut.

Hippocrates, who was known as the Father of Medicine said "All disease begins in the gut". He also said "Bad digestion is the root of all evil". There is a lot of truth in those statements.

The importance of stomach acid

When they think of stomach acid, most people consider it to be something bad; something that can cause heartburn and that should be reduced. Nothing can be further from the truth. Good, high levels of stomach acid are critical for optimum health.

Firstly though, before we even get to the stomach, we must mention that digestion begins in your mouth. How well and how thoroughly you chew your food will have an enormous impact on how well you extract the nutrients from your meal, and whether or not you'll be promoting the overgrowth of bad gut bugs. If you end up with undigested food in your small intestine, you're providing food for bacteria and yeast and leaving yourself wide open to developing SIBO. This can be a direct cause of leaky gut syndrome and nutrient deficiencies.

Once you've swallowed your food, it makes its way into your stomach. The cells of your stomach produce hydrochloric acid and the digestive enzyme called pepsin. Stomach acid and the enzyme pepsin are especially important for breaking down protein into its building blocks, called amino acids. It is also necessary for mineral absorption. Your stomach cells produce a type of molecule called intrinsic factor, which is critical for vitamin B12 absorption lower down in your small intestine. People with digestive problems or autoimmune disease are often low in vitamin B12.

When the acidic contents of your stomach make their way into the first part of your small intestine (called the duodenum), the acidity sends signals to your pancreas, for it to release digestive enzymes. Signals are also sent to your gallbladder, triggering it to release bile into your small intestine. The presence of fat in your small intestine also acts as a trigger for bile release.

So you can see that if your stomach is not producing optimal levels of acid, it creates problems further down your digestive tract, as your pancreas and gallbladder will then not function optimally. If you do not break down the protein you've eaten into its building blocks, you may absorb large protein molecules into your bloodstream. This is not supposed to happen, but it does in people with low stomach acid and digestive enzyme deficiencies. The large protein fragments are recognised by your immune system as foreign molecules, and you're then at high risk of developing a food allergy or intolerance. Low stomach acid is very common in people with allergic conditions such as eczema, asthma, hay fever and sinusitis. If these allergies are allowed to persist for years, it raises the risk of autoimmune disease later in life.

An inability to digest protein properly due to low stomach acid can also lead to amino acid deficiencies. Amino acids are necessary for neurotransmitter (brain chemical) production.

Impaired neurotransmitter production can lead to depression, anxiety or insomnia. Stomach acid is also a brilliant disinfectant; it helps to prevent the overgrowth of bacteria and fungus inside the stomach, and also further down in the small intestine. People with SIBO (Small Intestinal Bacterial Overgrowth) are almost always low in stomach acid. Producing adequate stomach acid also helps to protect you against food poisoning and gastroenteritis.

Symptoms of inadequate stomach acid

- Abdominal bloating.
- Flatulence.
- Burping.
- Eczema.
- Heartburn and/or reflux.
- Weak, splitting finger nails or vertical ridges on the nails.
- Weak, splitting hair and lacklustre hair.
- Vitamin B12 and/or iron deficiency.
- Food allergies.
- Gallbladder problems.
- Irritable bowel syndrome.
- Helicobacter pylori infection. This bug suppresses your ability to manufacture hydrochloric acid, in an attempt to survive inside your stomach.
- Bad breath.
- After age 50, stomach acid production sharply declines.

Antacids and medication for reflux and heartburn
suppress stomach acid production, and this has terrible
consequences for digestion and overall immune health

Most people think that heartburn and reflux are caused by too much stomach acid, but the reverse is true in the vast majority of cases. Most people with heartburn or reflux suffer with food intolerance because they haven't been digesting their food well for many years. Most people with these conditions also suffer with Small Intestinal Bacterial Overgrowth (SIBO). An inability to digest fermentable carbohydrates (FODMAPs) can create overgrowth of bacteria in the small intestine. This bacteria produce high levels of hydrogen gas. Hydrogen gas is actually a preferred fuel source for Helicobacter pylori[37].

The excess gas also raises the pressure inside the stomach and puts pressure on the lower oesophageal valve. This raises the risk of heartburn or reflux.

High levels of hydrogen gas in the intestines is also associated with infection with harmful bacteria such as Salmonella, E. coli and Campylobacter jejuni. These nasties are the leading cause of bacterial diarrhea. Foods high in certain types of fiber and starch, (such as FODMAPs) promote increased hydrogen production in people with SIBO. So does wheat. Therefore all those foods raise the risk of Helicobacter pylori infection. If you currently or previously had a Helicobacter pylori infection, we recommend you follow the stage 2 eating plan in chapter six.

Potential causes of low stomach acid

- Stress or anxiety. Your digestive system doesn't function well if you eat while upset
- Being over 50 years of age
- Acid suppressing medication typically given for heartburn or reflux or a peptic ulcer

- Nutrient deficiencies, particularly B vitamins and zinc
- Digestive diseases such as celiac disease or inflammatory bowel disease
- Infection with harmful bacteria or parasites

How to increase stomach acid and improve digestion

- If you are taking an antacid or other medication to block stomach acid, you may want to find a doctor or naturopath who can help you uncover food sensitivities or digestive problems that are causing you to suffer with reflux or heartburn. Following the stage 2 eating plan in chapter six may also eliminate these symptoms and eliminate the need for this medication.

- Try not to drink a lot of fluid with your meals because it dilutes digestive enzymes. Drink water and other beverages between meals.

- Try to eat in a calm and relaxed manner, and chew your food thoroughly.

- Find out if you have SIBO and take steps to treat it.

- Apple cider vinegar is brilliant for increasing stomach acid. Place 2 tablespoons of apple cider vinegar in ¼ mug of warm water and sip it 10 minutes before meals. If the vinegar feels uncomfortable going down, or burns you, drink it immediately before eating.

- Use lemon or lime juice as a dressing on your salads, along with a healthy oil such as olive oil, macadamia nut oil, avocado oil or coconut oil.

The most effective way of increasing stomach acid is to take a betaine hydrochloride (betaine HCL) supplement. This is essentially stomach acid in pill form. This usually works brilliantly for eliminating or reducing the symptoms of stomach acid deficiency listed earlier. It is excellent for helping you to extract more nutrients from your meals and supplements.

Doses in supplement form typically vary between 150 and 750 milligrams. Often betaine hydrochloride will be combined with pepsin (protein digesting enzyme) or other digestive enzymes in the same capsule.

Instructions for taking betaine hydrochloride supplements:

- Only take this supplement if you're going to be eating a significant quantity of protein. Therefore, if you're having a quick breakfast on the run of a banana and a few almonds, you wouldn't take a betaine supplement then.

- Take the supplement immediately before you start eating, or after you've had a few mouthfulls of food. Never take it on an empty stomach.

- Do not take betaine hydrochloride supplements if you are taking high dose corticosteroids (20mg or above), antacids or NSAIDs (Non-Steroidal Anti-inflammatory Drugs such as aspirin, ibuprofen, naproxen or diclofenac).

- Do not take betaine hydrochloride if you have a stomach or gastric ulcer.

The importance of bile

Bile is made in your liver and stored in your gallbladder. Your gallbladder squirts some bile into your small intestine whenever you eat a meal that contains some fat. There are cells in your small intestine that detect the presence of fat in food you've eaten and they secrete a hormone called cholecystokinin (CCK for short), which causes your gallbladder to contract. People with an irritated or inflamed gut lining often don't produce enough CCK and, therefore, their gallbladder isn't stimulated to contract properly.

This can leave stale bile behind in the gallbladder, raising the risk of stones in the gallbladder or inflammation of the gallbladder.

People with celiac disease and people with long term
bowel problems like irritable bowel syndrome are at
greater risk of developing gallbladder problems

If there are stones in the gallbladder, or other gallbladder conditions, not enough bile will be secreted into the small intestine for efficient fat digestion. Bile helps to break large fat globules into much smaller ones, so they can be broken down into fatty acids by digestive enzymes from the pancreas and intestine. Bile is also necessary for the proper digestion of fat soluble vitamins, including vitamins A, K, E and D. People with autoimmune disease are often low in these nutrients.

Ox bile supplements

You can purchase bile in capsule form. The bile comes from cows. It is purified and works very well at supplementing your own body's production of bile if it's inadequate. You may need an ox bile supplement if you have a gallbladder or liver problem, or if your autoimmune disease specifically affects your digestive organs or liver.

Anyone who feels like they don't digest fats well, and suffers with symptoms like bloating, burping, floating stools, very smelly stools or diarrhea after an oily meal would benefit from ox bile. If you take a vitamin D supplement but your blood level of vitamin D is still low, you'd also benefit from ox bile.

You can find ox bile in supplement form on its own or combined with digestive enzymes. Typical doses range between 100 and 500 milligrams. You would only take ox bile with a meal that contains some fat. If you find that it gives you diarrhea, try cutting the dose down. Conversely, people who suffer with constipation may find that ox bile relieves it for them.

The importance of digestive enzymes

Digestive enzymes are another component of a healthy and efficient digestive system. The bulk of the digestive enzymes in your body are made by your pancreas. Lots of things can impair adequate enzyme production, including stress, low stomach acid, inflammation of the pancreas due to gallbladder problems, dysbiosis or other factors. Everyone would benefit from taking a digestive enzymes supplement because they help you extract as much nutrition from your foods and supplements as possible, plus they ensure you don't leave undigested food behind, to act as food for bad gut bugs.

There are three main types of digestive enzymes:

- Amylase, which is a carbohydrate digesting enzyme.

- Protease, which digests protein.

- Lipase, which digests fat.

You can buy digestive enzymes that come from plants or animals. The ones derived from animals come from pig or cow pancreas or stomach. These enzymes are particularly good at helping you digest protein and fat. Plant derived enzymes are usually derived from fungi, although the final product is purified and is consequently free of fungi. Plant derived enzymes are particularly good at helping you digest carbohydrates from fruit and vegetables. If you experience bloating, burping, flatulence, irritable bowel syndrome, or you have celiac disease, you would greatly benefit from taking digestive enzymes.

If you have Small Intestinal Bacterial Overgrowth (SIBO), you need to take digestive supplements

Having poor digestion greatly increases your risk of developing an overgrowth of bacteria in your small intestine. Once you've developed an overgrowth, your digestion will deteriorate, which fosters a worsening of bacterial overgrowth. It's a vicious cycle.

Apart from the pancreas, the lining of your small intestine also produces some digestive enzymes. These are referred to as brush border enzymes. If the lining has become inflamed for whatever reason (SIBO is a common reason), you will not be producing adequate levels of enzymes anymore. It gets worse; the bacteria in the intestine of someone with SIBO actually degrade your digestive enzymes, and inhibit them from working. Protein degrading bacterial enzymes called proteinases break down your pancreatic and brush border enzymes, rendering them inactive.

Bacteria can also uncouple vitamin B12 bound with intrinsic factor, inhibiting you from being able to absorb vitamin B12 properly. Lastly, bacteria can deconjugate (break down) your bile salts from your gallbladder, interfering with your ability to digest fats and fat soluble vitamins. Small intestinal bacterial overgrowth is a significant problem in a large number of people with autoimmune disease, and it can be a major hurdle in trying to restore your digestive health and overall immune health.

The impact of autoimmune disease on liver health

The liver always suffers whenever there is autoimmune disease. If you have done some reading about autoimmune disease on the internet, you have probably already learned the importance of overcoming leaky gut, and the healing benefits of bone broth and fermented foods. These topics are getting a great deal of attention in the media and internet health community and that's wonderful. Unfortunately the liver is not getting enough attention.

If you have an autoimmune disease, you must make it a priority to improve the health of your liver

Autoimmune hepatitis, primary sclerosing cholangitis and primary biliary cirrhosis are three fairly common autoimmune diseases that affect the liver. They are serious diseases that can lead to liver scarring (cirrhosis) and sometimes even liver failure. However, every autoimmune disease will affect your liver, mainly through a leaky gut.

An excessively permeable intestinal lining (leaky gut) is present to varying degrees in all autoimmune conditions. When wastes, toxins and bacteria leak through the gut wall, where do they go? Straight to your liver. There is one main vein (the hepatic portal vein) that takes all blood from the gastrointestinal tract to the liver. Ordinarily this is a good thing because this blood is extremely rich in nutrients. Your liver is the hardest working organ in your body and it has a high need for nutrients. Your liver is also designed to trap any bacteria or foreign matter that may have escaped through the gut, preventing it from spreading to the rest of your body.

If your gut is toxic and leaky, your liver will quickly become overwhelmed. There are specialised cells inside your liver called Kupffer cells. They are a type of white blood cell called a macrophage; it comes from the Greek words "big eater"! The job of a macrophage is to engulf foreign matter, a lot like Pac Man. Macrophages contain enzymes that enable them to digest the debris or toxins they've swallowed.

If your gut is leaky, the high level of wastes arriving at your liver will trigger a great deal of inflammation inside your liver. One of the most harmful substances to travel from the gut to the liver is lipopolysaccharide. This is a type of endotoxin. It is a substance found in the cell wall of gram negative bacteria in the gut. If you have an overgrowth of bad bacteria in your gut, and if your gut is leaky, high levels of endotoxins will be arriving at your liver all the time.

Endotoxins stimulate Kupffer cells to produce high levels of inflammatory chemicals called cytokines. Some examples include interleukin 6 (IL6), Tumour Necrosis Factor alpha, and interleukin 1. These inflammatory chemicals are responsible for a lot of the symptoms of autoimmune disease, such as fatigue, pain, oedema and redness of the skin. They also affect your mood and cognitive abilities, promoting foggy head, poor memory, depression or anxiety. Lipopolysaccharide is a known pyrogen, meaning it can induce a fever. A mild fever unrelated to an infection is a very common symptom of autoimmune disease, and it can cause poor quality, disturbed sleep.

Typically, the liver will eventually become inflamed and start producing high levels of free radicals known as superoxides. These molecules are highly damaging to your entire body and they accelerate your rate of ageing.

It is very common to see mildly elevated liver enzymes on a blood test result of a patient with autoimmune disease. We also sometimes see a fatty liver on ultrasound. The liver accumulates fat inside it as a side effect from all the inflammatory damage. A blood test will also often show elevated levels of inflammatory markers called C-reactive protein and ESR (Erythrocyte Sedimentation Rate). There is more information about these tests in chapter nine.

When the liver is inflamed and overworked, it is not able to cleanse and purify your bloodstream adequately

This leads to an accumulation of metabolic wastes and inflammatory chemicals in the bloodstream, chronically stressing the immune system. This can lead to a worsening of an autoimmune disease.

If you want to reverse autoimmune disease and restore your health, it's vital to look after your liver. Following either the stage 1 or stage 2 eating plan in chapter six will go a long way towards improving your liver health. There are also certain herbs and nutrients that are wonderful for helping to improve liver health, and therefore helping to reverse autoimmune disease. They include St Mary's thistle, selenium and n-acetyl cysteine.. You can find these in LivaTone Plus. See www.liverdoctor.com for more information.

Chapter Five

Problematic foods for anyone with autoimmune disease

In chapter six you'll find practical information about the type of diet we recommend for healing autoimmune disease. We've included lists of the foods to eat and the foods to avoid, as well as meal ideas. We think it's important you understand the reasoning behind these diet guidelines. There are quite a few foods to avoid, and restrictive diets are always challenging. We believe if you understand the reasons why certain foods must be avoided, you'll be more motivated to stick with the diet.

The diet to heal autoimmune disease is designed to:

- Eliminate foods that promote a leaky gut by irritating and inflaming the intestines.

- Increase foods that heal the gut.

- Increase nutrient dense foods to help correct nutritional deficiencies.

- Support healthy liver function.

- Remove artificial additives in foods.

- Avoid foods that contain added sugar.

- Remove the foods most likely to cause food allergies or sensitivities.

- People with Small Intestinal Bacterial Overgrowth (SIBO) need a diet that eliminates fermentable carbohydrates (i.e. FODMAPs).

That's quite an ambitious list, but there is good research to support these dietary strategies in the treatment of autoimmune disease, and we've been utilising them with excellent results in our patients for many years.

Remember, research has shown that having a leaky gut is a necessary precursor to developing an autoimmune disease

There are other factors as well, such as genetics and exposure to environmental chemicals, but leaky gut is a major one. You can't change your genes and you can't always move to another city, but you can change what you eat, and that alone will give you a major improvement in your health.

Please also remember that you can't feel whether you have a leaky gut or not just by assessing your digestive symptoms. Even if you never get any bloating or indigestion, you have a leaky gut if you have an autoimmune disease. It can take at least 6 months to heal a leaky gut, and much longer if your autoimmune disease attacks your digestive system, such as celiac disease, Crohn's disease or ulcerative colitis.

The problem with gluten and other grains

Your entire life, you've probably been told that grains are good for you and should form a major part of your diet. You've been led to believe you need grains for their fiber content, plus vitamins and minerals. Unfortunately, grains have the potential to cause harm to the digestive tract and immune system of some people. Specifically, they can cause or aggravate a leaky gut.

Grains are a very recent introduction into the human diet, and some people seem poorly adapted to consuming them. Our ancestors survived very well without them. If you think of traditional diets in many parts of the world, grains did not form a significant component. For example, the traditional Aboriginal diet, Inuit diet and Polynesian diet did not feature grains. Of course, humans would eat whatever they could find, and if grains were the only foods available at a point in time, they would have been eaten. However, vegetables, animal protein, fruits and nuts are far more nutrient dense than grains.

If you have an autoimmune disease, grains are not your friend. Grain free diets have gained popularity in recent years. For instance, the paleo diet is a grain free diet, and also popular low carb, high fat diets exclude grains. These diets are often labelled as fad diets in the media. For people with autoimmune disease they are not a fad; staying away from grains can enable significant health improvements. Fortunately you won't miss out on anything by excluding grains from your diet.

Every nutrient found in grains can be easily obtained from other foods

The nutrients that are present in grains are usually difficult to absorb because of certain substances referred to as "anti-nutrients". They are enzyme inhibitors and lectins that reduce your ability to digest and absorb the vitamins and minerals in grains. There is an excellent research paper published by Professor Loren Cordain of the Department of Exercise and Sport Science, Colorado State University, Fort Collins, Colo., USA titled "Cereal Grains: Humanity's Double Edged Sword". It is available to read for free in its entirety on the internet if you'd like more information about the potentially harmful health effects of grains.

Grains that contain gluten are the biggest problem for people with autoimmune disease, but other grains contain substances that can irritate the gut lining too. Therefore we recommend you avoid all gluten and also avoid gluten free grains, such as corn and rice. While trying to reverse an autoimmune disease, we also recommend you avoid grain-like foods such as quinoa and amaranth. Most people can eat those foods later on, once their health improves.

Grains are especially high in a type of protein called lectins. Lectins are present in most foods, but the types of lectins found in grains can be harmful to the intestines. The two worst lectins are prolamins (gluten is an example) and agglutinins (such as wheat germ agglutinin). Prolamins are very difficult for the human body to digest. Gluten is comprised of gliadins and glutenins. The human body actually cannot digest gluten. We don't make the enzymes necessary for breaking it apart. This is a problem because it means gluten can cross the intestinal lining intact, or partially digested. Gluten can also promote the overgrowth of harmful gut microbes, creating dysbiosis.

Lectins are a way plants protect themselves from attack by pests or predators. In nature, every living thing is just trying to survive. Because plants can't run away from a predator, they increase their chances of survival by producing toxins. The toxins are usually most concentrated in the seed of the grain, which is the part that people eat. Gluten is a lectin rich in the amino acid proline.

Lectins can either damage and kill the cells that line your intestines (called enterocytes) or cause spaces to open up between your intestinal cells. The resultant little holes in your intestines allow wastes and toxins to leak into your bloodstream; then you'll have a leaky gut. Recent research is showing that gluten seems to trigger the release of zonulin in people with autoimmune disease. Zonulin causes the gap junctions between intestinal cells to open up, creating a leaky gut. This was once thought to only apply to people with celiac disease, but research is uncovering the phenomenon in more and more autoimmune and inflammatory conditions.

If you want to heal a leaky gut, you'll have to stop eating all gluten and all wheat

Wheat germ agglutinin is present in the entire wheat plant, including wheat grass, so its essential to avoid that too. Gluten free grains also contain lectins, therefore you will not be able to eat gluten free bread, pasta or other gluten substitutes at the moment, if you want to reverse autoimmune disease.

Celiac disease is a serious autoimmune disease where the ingestion of gluten causes destruction to the lining of the small intestine. Every last trace of gluten must be removed from the diet in order to allow the intestines to heal. We would like to make it clear to you that you need to avoid eating gluten if you wish to heal autoimmune disease, even if you don't have celiac disease, gluten intolerance or wheat allergy.

Gluten increases intestinal permeability in celiacs and non-celiacs by triggering the production of the protein called zonulin[38].

Zonulin opens the tight junctions between endothelial cells in the gut. That means it creates spaces between gut cells, which allow gut toxins into the bloodstream. People with autoimmune disease, and people with inflammatory diseases have been found to produce high levels of zonulin in response to gluten ingestion. Gluten can also damage intestinal cells while getting absorbed into them, leading to their death.

What is gluten?

Gluten is a protein found in some grains, including wheat, rye, barley, triticale, spelt and kamut. Oats don't contain gluten; they contain a protein called avenin. It's extremely similar to gluten though, and most people with gluten sensitivity react to it in the same destructive way as to gluten.

Gluten is a gluey substance; it gives dough its elasticity and enables bread to become light and fluffy. If you've ever made your own bread or pizza dough, you'll know how stretchy the dough becomes. That's courtesy of gluten. If you tried the same recipe with rice flour you'd have a disaster.

Speaking of rice, you may have noticed glutenous rice for sale at the supermarket. There is no gluten in rice; this term just describes the sticky nature of the rice. Although rice is gluten free, it needs to be avoided during the eating plan in this book because it is capable of causing intestinal inflammation in some people with autoimmune disease. You will probably be able to eat rice once you have reached a state of health you are happy with.

Wheat fiber can cause vitamin D deficiency

The fiber in wheat can reduce the ability of your body to absorb vitamin D from supplements, and can leave you vitamin D deficient despite plentiful sun exposure.

Epidemiological studies conducted in the 1980s found that vitamin D deficiency and rickets were more prevalent in people who ate a lot of wholegrain bread, compared to those that didn't. Therefore researchers decided to conduct a study comparing blood vitamin D levels of individuals who ate a normal diet, to those who supplemented their diet with 60 grams of wheat bran each day.

After 30 days, those eating wheat bran had significantly lower blood vitamin D levels. The researchers believe that wheat bran reduces enterohepatic circulation of vitamin D (i.e. recycling of vitamin D between the gut and liver). Wheat bran also increases vitamin D elimination via the stool[39].

The insoluble fiber in wheat, and probably other grains as well, impairs the absorption of fat soluble vitamins such as vitamin D. Another good reason to avoid grains.

Harmful effects of lectins

In 1999 an article appeared in the British Medical Journal called **Do dietary lectins cause disease?** It is a brief yet very interesting summary of the harmful effects of some lectins in some people.

We have reproduced the majority of the article below:

Do dietary lectins cause disease?

The evidence is suggestive - and raises interesting possibilities for treatment

David L J Freed, Allergist BMJ 1999 Apr 17;318 (7190):1023-1024[40]

In 1988 a hospital launched a "healthy eating day" in its staff canteen at lunchtime. One dish contained red kidney beans, and 31 portions were served.

At 3 pm one of the customers, a surgical registrar, vomited in theatre. Over the next four hours 10 more customers suffered profuse vomiting, some with diarrhea.

All had recovered by next day. No pathogens were isolated from the food, but the beans contained an abnormally high concentration of the lectin phytohaemagglutinin.[1] Lectins are carbohydrate binding proteins present in most plants, especially seeds and tubers like cereals, potatoes, and beans. Until recently their main use was as histology and blood transfusion reagents, but in the past two decades we have realised that many lectins are (a) toxic, inflammatory, or both; (b) resistant to cooking and digestive enzymes; and (c) present in much of our food.[2] It is thus no surprise that they sometimes cause "food poisoning." But the really disturbing finding came with the discovery in 1989 that some food lectins get past the gut wall and deposit themselves in distant organs.[3,4] So do they cause real life diseases?

Wheat gliadin, which causes celiac disease, contains a lectin like substance that binds to human intestinal mucosa,[6] and this has been debated as the "celiac disease toxin" for over 20 years.[7] But celiac disease is already managed by gluten avoidance, so nothing would change were the lectin hypothesis proved. On the other hand, wheat lectin also binds to glomerular capillary walls, mesangial cells, and tubules of human kidney and (in rodents) binds IgA and induces IgA mesangial deposits. This suggests that in humans IgA nephropathy might be caused or aggravated by wheat lectin; indeed a trial of gluten avoidance in children with this disease reported reduced proteinuria and immune complex levels.[8]

Of particular interest is the implication for autoimmune diseases. Lectins stimulate class II HLA antigens on cells that do not normally display them, such as pancreatic islet and thyroid cells.[9] The islet cell determinant to which cytotoxic autoantibodies bind in insulin dependent diabetes mellitus is the disaccharide N-acetyl lactosamine,[10] which must bind tomato lectin if present and probably also the lectins of wheat, potato, and peanuts. This would result in islet cells expressing both class II HLA antigens and foreign antigen together—a sitting duck for autoimmune attack.

Certain foods (wheat, soya) are indeed diabetogenic in genetically susceptible mice.[11] Insulin dependent diabetes therefore is another potential lectin disease and could possibly be prevented by prophylactic oligosaccharides.

Another suspect lectin disease is rheumatoid arthritis. The normal human IgG molecule possesses carbohydrate side chains, which terminate with galactose. In rheumatoid arthritis much of the galactose is missing, so that the subterminal sugar—N-acetyl glucosamine—is exposed instead. These deficient IgG molecules feature strongly in the circulating immune complexes that cause fever and symptoms.[12] In diet responsive rheumatoid arthritis one of the commonest trigger foods is wheat, and wheat lectin is specific for N-acetyl glucosamine—the sugar that is normally hidden but exposed in rheumatoid arthritis. This suggests that N-acetyl glucosamine oligomers such as chitotetraose (derived from the chitin that forms crustacean shells) might be an effective treatment for diet associated rheumatoid arthritis. Interestingly, the health food trade has already siezed on N-acetyl glucosamine as an antiarthritic supplement.[13]

Among the effects observed in the small intestine of lectin fed rodents is stripping away of the mucous coat to expose naked mucosa and overgrowth of the mucosa by abnormal bacteria and protozoa.[14] Lectins also cause discharge of histamine from gastric mast cells,[15] which stimulates acid secretion. So the three main pathogenic factors for peptic ulcer—acid stimulation, failure of the mucous defence layer, and abnormal bacterial proliferation (Helicobacter pylori) are all theoretically linked to lectins. If true, blocking these effects by oligosaccharides would represent an attractive and more physiological treatment for peptic ulcer than suppressing stomach acid.

The mucus stripping effect of lectins[16] also offers an explanation for the anecdotal finding of many allergists that a "stone age diet," which eliminates most starchy foods and therefore most lectins, protects against common upper respiratory viral infections: without lectins in the throat the nasopharyngeal mucus lining would be more effective as a barrier to viruses.

But if we all eat lectins, why don't we all get insulin dependent diabetes, rheumatoid arthritis, IgA nephropathy, and peptic ulcers? Partly because of biological variation in the glycoconjugates that coat our cells and partly because these are protected behind a fine screen of sialic acid molecules, attached to the glycoprotein tips.[10] We should be safe. But the sialic acid molecules can be stripped off by the enzyme neuraminidase, present in several micro-organisms such as influenza viruses and streptococci. This may explain why diabetes and rheumatoid arthritis tend to occur as sequelae of infections. This facilitation of lectins by micro-organisms throws a new light on post-infectious diseases and makes the folklore cure of fasting during a fever seem sensible.

Alternative medicine popularisers are already publishing articles about dietary lectins,[17] often with more enthusiasm than caution, so patients are starting to ask about them and doctors need to be armed with facts. The same comment applies to entrepreneurs at the opposite end of the commercial spectrum. Many lectins are powerful allergens, and prohevein, the principal allergen of rubber latex, is one. It has been engineered into transgenic tomatoes for its fungistatic properties,[18] so we can expect an outbreak of tomato allergy in the near future among latex sensitive individuals. Dr Arpad Pusztai lost his job for publicising concerns of this type (20 February, p 483).

Here is a summary of the problems with lectins:

- They can increase gut permeability by stripping away the protective mucous lining of your intestines.
- Lectins promote the overgrowth of harmful bacteria and protozoa in the intestines.
- They raise inflammation in your body.
- They are indigestible. Humans don't make the necessary enzymes to digest lectins.
- Lectins bind to carbohydrates. That means they can bind to components of your own body, such as your intestinal lining. This can trigger an inflammatory immune attack on the gut lining in some individuals.
- Lectins reduce your ability to absorb minerals from the foods or supplements you've ingested.
- Lectins can be absorbed through your gut, enter your bloodstream and then get deposited in distant organs or tissues. This can trigger an autoimmune response in various parts of your body.
- The research linking lectins with autoimmune disease is strongest for type 1 diabetes, rheumatoid arthritis and IgA nephropathy (kidney disease).

- They may promote the growth of Helicobacter pylori in the stomach and raise the risk of peptic ulcers.

- Lectins are found in many foods, and not everyone who eats them will ever develop an autoimmune disease. You need to have a genetic susceptibility, and it appears that certain infections may be triggers for lectin-induced autoimmune disease. These are common infections, such as the viruses that cause the flu and streptococcal bacterial infections.

The problem with legumes

Legumes are plants that produce a pod with seeds inside. We refer to the edible seeds as legumes. Common examples include lentils, peas, chickpeas, beans, soybeans and peanuts.

Legumes contain fairly high levels of protein, minerals and fiber. At least on paper they do. The problem is these nutrients are fairly difficult to absorb because of various substances present inside them.

Legumes are unsuitable if you're trying to reverse autoimmune disease for the following reasons:

- They contain lectins, as already mentioned.

- They contain enzyme inhibitors, particularly trypsin inhibitors. Enzyme inhibitors prevent your own digestive enzymes from working, thereby compromising your digestion.

- Legumes are very high in FODMAPs. This is a problem for anyone suffering with small intestinal bacterial overgrowth or irritable bowel syndrome. The undigested starch can provide food for harmful gut microbes.

- They contain saponins, which are substances that resist digestion and increase intestinal permeability.

- Soybeans are a legume that contains goitrogens, which are substances that reduce your ability to absorb iodine. This is particularly a problem for people with a thyroid condition.

The problem with dairy products

If you are trying to overcome an autoimmune disease, we strongly recommend you exclude dairy products from your diet for several reasons.

Dairy products refers to cow's milk and any foods made from or containing cow's milk. We also recommend you avoid consuming milk from other animals such as goats, sheep and water buffalo. They are certainly less problematic than cow's milk, and you may be able to introduce them into your diet at a later stage. A2 cow's milk is also often better tolerated. If you really miss milk and yogurt, you can try introducing the A2 variety into your diet once your autoimmune disease is under control and you are happy with your state of health.

Dairy products are highly inflammatory foods that irritate the gut and immune system

If you are trying to overcome an autoimmune disease, you need to reduce inflammation and heal your gut. The main problem with dairy products is caused by the protein called casein. Casein is a highly allergenic protein and many people develop a sensitivity to it. Antibodies to beta-casein are present in large numbers of people with autoimmune disease. They have been found to be most common in people with type 1 diabetes, celiac disease and latent autoimmune diabetes in adults (LADA).[41]

It is thought that via molecular mimicry, the immune system of someone with a casein intolerance can eventually start producing antibodies against their own organs or tissues. The pancreas seems to be the most vulnerable organ. A lot of research has been done on the relationship between dairy products and type 1 diabetes. It is known that early introduction of cow's milk into an infant's diet (before six months of age), short duration of breastfeeding, or not being breastfed at all are all risk factors. [42]

Cow's milk contains a lot more casein than human milk does (85 percent versus 25 percent), and the majority of it is beta-casein. Antibodies to beta-casein are very common in type 1 diabetics, and so too is enhanced proliferation of lymphocytes (white blood cells) in response to beta-casein; meaning dairy products are highly irritating to the immune system of people with this autoimmune disease. There is also a strong relationship between casein sensitivity and schizophrenia. Some forms of schizophrenia are thought to be autoimmune. Research has shown an association between production of bovine casein antibodies and subsequent diagnosis of schizophrenia.[43]

There are other problems with dairy products:

- Dairy allergy is extremely common and typically manifests are eczema, dermatitis, asthma, hay fever or sinusitis. Most people with a dairy allergy do not go on to develop type 1 diabetes or schizophrenia, but regularly eating any food you have a sensitivity to will irritate your immune system and inflame your gut, creating a leaky gut.

- Lactose intolerance is a problem for a significant percentage of the world's population. Actually on a global scale, not being able to digest lactose is more common than being able to digest it. Only approximately 15 percent of caucasians are lactose intolerant. This figure jumps to between 50 and 100 percent of asians, hispanics, african americans and native americans. These figures relate to lactose intolerance, while a milder form of intolerance called lactose maldigestion is far more common.[44] This is a problem because lactose is a fermentable carbohydrate; meaning if you are not digesting it thoroughly it will provide food for potentially harmful gut microbes and may contribute to SIBO (Small Intestinal Bacterial Overgrowth). Please do not consume lactose free milk, however, as it still contains casein.

- The proteins in cow's milk are potential cross-reactors to gluten. That means people with celiac disease or non-celiac gluten sensitivity may mount an immune response to dairy products and their immune system starts behaving as though they're consuming gluten.

- Dairy products increase mucus production. That's bad news if you're a singer, suffer with asthma, have a cold or flu, but it's also bad for your digestive tract. Excess mucus in the gut can hinder nutrient absorption.

- Milk contains growth promoting hormones. This makes sense because in nature only creatures that are growing rapidly consume it (i.e. infants). Consuming dairy products can raise your blood level of insulin-like growth factor 1 and higher levels are associated with a raised risk of breast, prostate and colorectal cancer. As adults, we are no longer growing, hence there is no requirement to consume dairy products. All of the nutrients found in milk can be easily obtained through other foods.

You may consume ghee (clarified butter) because it contains negligible levels of lactose or casein. In fact, ghee can be very beneficial if you are suffering with inflammatory bowel disease such as Crohn's disease or ulcerative colitis. This is because ghee is high in a type of beneficial short chain fatty acid called butyrate. Butyrate can calm down inflammation in the intestines. A study titled *"Oral butyrate for mildly to moderately active Crohn's disease"* stated the following:

"Oral butyrate is safe and well tolerated, and may be effective in inducing clinical improvement/remission in Crohn's disease. These data indicate the need for a large investigation to extend the present findings, and suggest that butyrate may exert its action through downregulation of NF-kappaB and IL-1beta."[45]

Nightshade vegetables

Vegetables in the nightshade family include tomatoes, eggplant, peppers (bell pepper, paprika and chilli), goji berries and potatoes. Sweet potatoes are in a different botanical family and the information that follows does not apply to them.

The botanical name of the nightshade plants is solanaceae. Nightshade vegetables are problematic for some people with autoimmune disease because they contain a type of saponin called glycoalkaloids. There are many different types of saponins and they are found in all plants, including grains and legumes. Some specific saponins can irritate the gut lining and contribute to leaky gut.

Saponins have detergent-like properties and they are designed to protect plants against consumption by insects, by dissolving the cell membranes of the insects, thereby killing them. Saponins have the ability to create holes in the surface membrane of your intestinal cells (enterocytes), thereby allowing a variety of substances and wastes in your intestine to leak into your cells. This causes damage to the intestinal cells and, hence, increases intestinal permeability, contributing to the development of a leaky gut.

The saponins in nightshade vegetables are also strong immune system irritants. They are adjuvants, meaning they stimulate the immune system. Tomato lectin has actually been investigated for use in intranasal vaccines because it has the ability to stimulate antibody production.

Not everyone with an autoimmune disease needs to avoid all nightshade vegetables. Sensitivity varies among individuals. The people who benefit most from their elimination are those with joint disease or muscle disease, such as rheumatoid arthritis and other autoimmune diseases that affect the joints, and also fibromyalgia. There is research to show that potato glycoalkaloids cause a leaky gut and aggravate inflammatory bowel disease (Crohn's disease and ulcerative colitis). There is an interesting study published in the journal Inflammatory Bowel Disease titled *"Potato glycoalkaloids adversely affect intestinal permeability and aggravate inflammatory bowel disease".* The article states the following:

"Disruption of epithelial barrier integrity is important in the initiation and cause of inflammatory bowel disease (IBD). Glycoalkaloids, solanine (S), and chaconine (C) are naturally present in potatoes, can permeabilize cholesterol-containing membranes, and lead to disruption of epithelial barrier integrity. Frying potatoes concentrates glycoalkaloids. Interestingly, the prevalence of inflammatory bowel disease is highest in countries where fried potatoes consumption is highest." [46]

> *If joint or muscle pain is a feature of your autoimmune disease, please avoid nightshade vegetables, and if you suffer with inflammatory bowel disease, please avoid nightshade vegetables*

If you have been following one of our eating plans in chapter six for more than three months and haven't experienced significant improvements, you may want to try eliminating this group of foods from your diet for a month to see if it helps.

The problem with eggs

Eggs are a highly nutritious food and very healthy for most people. They certainly won't raise your cholesterol or cause heart disease. Unfortunately eggs are one of the most common food allergens and may need to be avoided temporarily by those trying to reverse autoimmune disease.

The problem is usually caused by the egg white, rather than the yolk. Egg white contains enzymes designed to protect the yolk against microbial attack while the chicken embryo is developing. These are protein digesting enzymes and are referred to as lysozymes. Different types of lysozymes are found extensively in nature and they are even produced by your own body; they are present in your saliva, mucus and tears, to help prevent infections. Lysozymes are resistant to acid and heat, therefore are not destroyed by cooking eggs or by our stomach acid.

The specific lysozymes in eggs have the ability to bind tightly with other proteins in egg white, and these protein complexes cannot be digested by our digestive enzymes. Therefore, the lysozyme protein complex travels through your gut, resisting digestion. If you have an autoimmune disease, you have probably had a leaky gut for some time. A leaky gut allows large protein molecules in the gut to be absorbed across the gut wall, into the bloodstream. This triggers an immune response and eventually you can start to form antibodies against egg white proteins.

Interestingly, lysozymes are also able to bind with bacterial proteins from the bacteria that normally live in your gut. These bacterial proteins can make their way across the gut wall if you have a leaky gut. Therefore, the various proteins that piggyback on the lysozyme and cross the intestinal lining can trigger an immune response and antibody production. Therefore, in time, you can develop an egg allergy. The bacterial proteins that make their way across the gut wall can chronically stimulate the immune system and eventually trigger autoantibody production through the process of molecular mimicry.

There are varying degrees of egg sensitivity and a plethora of different symptoms a person could experience

Egg sensitivity can produce immediate, obvious symptoms such as eczema, wheezing, indigestion or a headache, or the response may be delayed by several days and include symptoms such as acne, nausea, irritable bowel syndrome or disturbed sleep. The most reliable way to find out if eggs are adversely affecting you is to exclude them from your diet for six weeks, monitor how you feel; reintroduce them and monitor how you feel.

Nuts and seeds

Nuts and seeds are healthy foods that are high in minerals, fiber and good fats, and you can include them in your diet. Please remember that peanuts are legumes, so they should be avoided. The types of nuts we are referring to in this section are tree nuts.

There are a couple of potential problems with nuts; they are a very common cause of food allergy or intolerance, and they can be difficult to digest. Some people find that nuts make them feel bloated, give them gas or cause irritable bowel syndrome. If you do eat nuts, it's best to keep your consumption low; sprinkle them on a salad, have them with breakfast or as a snack.

You can make nuts easier to digest by soaking them first. This process is commonly referred to as activating nuts. The nuts are soaked overnight in the fridge in fresh water. The next morning drain and rinse them. You can eat them like that straight away or dehydrate them in the oven at the very lowest heat or in a food dehydrator. Please be aware that you should consume the nuts shortly after soaking them because they become prone to mould growth. Only nuts with a skin require soaking, therefore macadamia nuts, cashews and pine nuts don't require activating.

In the past, the media has had a field day making fun of activated nuts and referring to it as a fad. The truth is there's nothing new about this process. Several cultures, particularly in the Middle East have soaked nuts before consuming them because it's known to make the nuts more easily digested. It's a custom that has been handed down for many generations.

Most nuts are fairly high in FODMAPs, therefore can aggravate small intestinal bacterial overgrowth by acting as food for undesirable gut microbes. Therefore, people with irritable bowel syndrome or small intestinal bacterial overgrowth may need to avoid them temporarily.

The other problem with nuts is their potential to cause food allergy or intolerance. Like with any food, discovering a nut allergy can be a tricky process, as the symptoms aren't always obvious. An elimination diet is really the best method of uncovering hidden food sensitivities. We have found that sensitivity to almonds is the most common of all nuts, probably because they are the most commonly consumed nut, and a lot of people use almond meal for baking gluten free muffins, bread, etcetera. Therefore, our advice while following the eating plan in chapter six is to eat nuts you don't often consume, as you are less likely to have a sensitivity to them. Macadamia nuts, pecans and pine nuts are some examples.

Harmful effects of sugar on the immune system

Consuming sugar raises inflammation in your body for a number of reasons. Sugar itself is inflammatory and it increases the production of inflammatory chemicals such as cytokines in your body. A high carbohydrate meal causes more postprandial (post meal) inflammation than a low carbohydrate meal. This is especially true for anyone who is overweight (particularly around the torso), suffers with diabetes, polycystic ovarian syndrome or insulin resistance. The higher these inflammatory chemicals, the more pain and fatigue you are likely to experience.

Sugar is also detrimental because it acts like fertiliser for bad bugs and bad yeast in your intestines

Every time you eat sugar you are feeding the bad microbes in your gut. These bad microbes produce a host of inflammatory chemicals that make you feel rotten, and they inflame your gut lining, giving you a leaky gut. There are a number of ways to reduce levels of harmful microbes in your gut, which we explain in chapter four. One of the best ways is to simply starve them of their food supply; and that means don't eat sugar.

Chapter Six

Foods to eat to heal autoimmune disease

Food is powerful. It has the power to make you very ill or very healthy. Food is also something that's under your control. There are a lot factors that probably contributed towards the development of your autoimmune disease - genes, environmental chemicals, stressful life events. Unfortunately, you had very little control over those factors. Luckily, you do have enormous control over what you eat. Even if you've inherited terrible genes from your parents, the food you eat determines how your genes function. You don't have to suffer with the same health problems as your family.

The eating plan in this book is very restrictive. There are a lot of foods to cut out. It's stressful to have to make big changes to your diet.

> *You've probably been cooking and eating the way you do for a long time because it works for you. Well, the fact is, it's not really working for your body. If you want different health outcomes, you're going to have to change what you eat!*

Many of the foods we ask you to exclude are typically considered to be healthy foods. They can be healthy, for lots of people. They're probably just not appropriate for you to eat if you want to reverse your autoimmune disease. We have explained the reasons why certain foods are problematic for people with autoimmune disease in chapter five. Please read that chapter thoroughly. If you can have a good understanding of why you're avoiding your favourite foods, you are much more likely to remain motivated and approach these diet changes from a positive state of mind.

The aim of our diet guidelines is for you to consume nutrient dense foods, to provide your body with optimal levels of vitamins, minerals and other nutrients required for good immune health and tissue healing. It is also critical to stop eating foods that inflame and irritate the gut lining. We'll start with listing all the foods you can eat, and later on you'll find a summary of the foods that need to be avoided for the time being.

Vegetables

Why they're beneficial

We all agree that vegetables are good for you; that's something every diet plan has in common. Vegetables are a wonderful source of vitamins, minerals, antioxidants and fiber. The fiber acts as a prebiotic, providing food for the beneficial microbes in your gut. The nutrients in vegetables help support healthy liver function; they enable your liver to be a better detoxifier.

Vegetables are also a wonderful source of phytonutrients. Phytonutrients are very tiny metabolites in foods, and they perform a number of different medicinal functions in the body. So far, approximately 10 thousand of them have been identified in our food supply. We find them in fruits, vegetables, nuts, seeds, whole grains, legumes, herbs, and spices. Most phytonutrients are pigments, therefore are abundant in brightly coloured vegetables and fruits, but not all phytonutrients have colours. There are some that are pigmented and some that are not.

There are three categories of vegetables and we'd like you to consume some from each category every day. The three categories are:

- Leafy vegetables - e.g. bok choy, spinach, lettuce, fresh herbs.
- Brightly coloured vegetables - e.g. pumpkin, carrots, red bell pepper
- Sulfur rich vegetables - e.g. onion, garlic, broccoli, cabbage

Leafy vegetables are an excellent source of B vitamins, especially folate (folic acid). B vitamins are necessary for energy production, red blood cell production, as well as healthy mood and cognitive function. Brightly coloured red, orange and yellow vegetables contain beta carotene and other carotenoids. Some of these are precursors to vitamin A, and others act as antioxidants in the body. Carotenoids help to keep your eyes healthy and improve night vision. Dark green vegetables are also a source of carotenoids, but the deep green colour of chlorophyll overrides the orange pigments.

Vegetables are a rich source of vitamin C, which supports healthy immune system function, strong and healthy collagen, as well as reducing inflammation. Green vegetables are a good source of vitamin K1. Good bacteria in your intestines convert it into the more potent vitamin K2. Vitamin K helps to strengthen bones and reduce the risk of cardiovascular disease. Vitamin K is also necessary for the production of myelin, therefore is helpful for all nerve problems, especially multiple sclerosis.[47]

Sulfur rich vegetables help your body to be more efficient at eliminating toxins, as they are required by your liver to carry out phase 2 detoxification. People with a leaky gut usually have sluggish liver function because the liver is greatly burdened by the toxins arriving from the gut. These vegetables contain the compound sulforaphane, which assists detoxification, reduces oxidative stress in the body and induces the production of glutathione.[48]

Sulfur is also required for producing collagen, which is what your connective tissue is made of. Additional sulfur can help anyone with a connective tissue disease (e.g. lupus), joint disease or skin disease. Vegetables high in sulfur include those in the onion and garlic family, as well as those in the cruciferous family (e.g. kale, cabbage, broccoli). If you have one of the mentioned health problems, you would benefit from additional sulfur in the form of MSM, which can be taken in supplement form combined with vitamin C and silica, known as Collagen Food.

Vegetables to eat

This is not a complete list; we have just given you some examples. If it's a vegetable, you can eat it, even if it doesn't appear on this list. Please vary your vegetable intake as much as possible; try new vegetables you've never eaten before.

Examples of vegetables to include in your diet:

- leafy vegetables - e.g. bok choy, spinach, silverbeet, endive
- cruciferous vegetables - e.g. broccoli, cauliflower, cabbage, kale, Brussels sprouts
- carrots
- beetroot
- zucchini
- cucumber
- radishes
- celery
- fresh herbs - e.g. parsley, basil, cilantro, arugula, dill, watercress
- turnip
- swede
- sweet potato
- pumpkin
- asparagus
- artichoke
- allium family vegetables - e.g. leek, garlic, onion, spring onion, chives
- snow peas

Vegetables to avoid

- Potatoes are best avoided by everyone with autoimmune disease because research has shown they can cause gut inflammation and joint inflammation.

- Nightshade vegetables may need to be avoided by some people - i.e. tomatoes, bell pepper, chilli, potatoes, paprika and eggplant.

- High FODMAP vegetables need to be avoided by people with Small Intestinal Bacterial Overgrowth. The stage 2 eating plan in this chapter is low FODMAP.

Fruit

Fruit is an excellent source of vitamins, antioxidants, phytonutrients and soluble fiber. Please include a variety of different fruits in your diet. It is best to limit your intake of fruit to two serving sizes per day for a couple of reasons:

- Fruit is fairly high in natural sugars (fructose and glucose). People with insulin resistance are sensitive to sugar and it tends to promote a rise in insulin and blood sugar, which raises inflammation. If consumed in high amounts, fructose can promote abdominal weight gain. This is the worst place to gain weight in terms of your health because fat cells here produce inflammatory chemicals.

- The fructose in fruit is a fermentable carbohydrate and it may cause bloating and other digestive problems for some people, and it may encourage the growth of harmful gut microbes. When glucose is present in greater or equal amounts than fructose (such as in bananas, melon and berries), the fructose is well absorbed across your intestinal wall. This is because glucose helps to carry fructose across the intestinal wall. However, if there's more fructose than glucose in a fruit (such as apples, pears and peaches), the additional fructose can linger in the gut and provide food for harmful gut bacteria (they ferment it). This is not an issue for everyone, but is common in people with poor digestion.

Good fruits to eat

- berries
- citrus fruits
- kiwifruit
- bananas
- melons
- cherries
- papaya
- mango
- apricots
- plums
- nectarines
- peaches

All other fruits are fine to consume, unless you need to follow a low FODMAP diet. See the stage 2 eating plan later in this chapter.

This is an interesting article that appeared in a UK newspaper about fruit (particularly bananas) being banned in a zoo in England. Yes fruit is healthy, but the kind of fruit we eat these days is very different to how fruit used to be.

If you've ever gone on a road trip through the south island of New Zealand and eaten wild Granny Smith apples growing on the side of the road, you'll know there's a world of difference. Traditional fruits were much smaller, very sour and very fibrous. The Granny Smith apples were almost like lemons!

Modern fruits have been bred to be big, sweet and very juicy (lower in fiber). Eating large amounts of fruit like that isn't in your best interest

Paignton Zoo monkeys banned from eating bananas

BBC online 14 January, 2014

Monkeys at a zoo have been banned from eating bananas because keepers say they are too sugary.

Paignton Zoo in Devon says giving monkeys bananas cultivated for humans is like giving them cake and chocolate.

Amy Plowman, head of conservation, said that is because they are too ripe for monkeys and can cause gastrointestinal problems.

Dr Plowman said it had not been too hard to wean the monkeys off bananas and give them vegetables instead.

She said: "Fruit cultivated for humans is much higher in sugar and much lower in protein and fiber than most wild fruit.

"It can also cause gastrointestinal problems as their stomachs are mostly adapted to eating fibrous foods with very low digestibility."

Bananas 'a treat'

She said monkeys had their banana intake reduced slowly.

A typical monkey diet now features lots of green leafy vegetables, smaller amounts of other vegetables and as much browse - leafy branches - as possible.

Animals do still get bananas if they are unwell and the keepers need to make sure they take medication.

Dr Plowman said: "Putting it in a piece of banana works really well, as it's such a treat now."

Senior head keeper of mammals Matthew Webb said: "Reducing the sugar in their diets has calmed them down and made their group more settled."

http://www.bbc.com/news/uk-england-devon-25728179

Animal protein

Seafood

You can eat all types of seafood. It is a rich source of complete protein, minerals and omega 3 essential fatty acids. Most fish is a good source of B vitamins. Oily fish like mackerel, salmon, sardines and herrings can be a good source of vitamin D and vitamin A. Wild seafood is higher in nutrients and lower in toxins than farmed seafood.

Most types of seafood are a reasonable source of minerals including iodine, phosphorus, potassium, and selenium. Canned fish such as salmon and sardines that contain bones that have softened during the canning process are a good source of calcium. Some shellfish, such as clams and oysters, are a good source of iron, zinc, magnesium and copper. Please see page 42 for guidance on which seafood to avoid because of high mercury levels. You can eat all other types of seafood that you enjoy. Please choose wild over farmed seafood.

Red meat and poultry

You can eat all types of poultry and all types of red meat. They are all an excellent source of easily digested complete protein. Complete protein means they contain all 21 essential amino acids (the building blocks of protein). They are also an excellent source of vitamins, minerals and healthy fats.

Red meat and poultry are an excellent source of iron, zinc, selenium, phosphorus and all the B group vitamins, including vitamin B12. Try to vary the types of red meat and poultry you consume. The eating plan we recommend in this book is really quite restrictive, so please don't make your diet even more restrictive than it needs to be. Perhaps you'd like to try spatchcock, kangaroo, goat, emu, wallaby or other animal protein you haven't tried before. You'll obtain a wider range of nutrients and the diet won't seem as monotonous.

If available and affordable, grass fed and finished meat and poultry is preferable. Ideally, the animals you eat would have as healthy a diet as possible, because while it's true that you are what you eat, it's also true that you are what you eat ate!

Ruminants (cows and sheep) are healthiest when they eat the foods their bodies were designed to eat - grass and some broad leafed plants. Their health suffers when they are fed foods their bodies were not adapted to eat, such as grains.

The fatty acid composition of grass fed meat is better than grain fed. There are more anti-inflammatory omega 3 fats in grass fed meat and less potentially inflammatory omega 6 fats. There is also more oleic acid; a monounsaturated fat found abundantly in olive oil. Grass fed animals are usually allowed to roam freely outside, which is not only healthier for the animals and gives them a better quality of life; their body fat contains some vitamin D because of their exposure to sunlight. By consuming them, you'll get more vitamin D in your diet.

An increasing number of butchers and supermarkets are selling grass fed meat because demand is growing. Fortunately, this means the price is coming down. You will probably be able to find grass fed meat at your local farmers' market. This is a great way to support your local farmers.

Does red meat cause cancer and heart disease?

Red meat has a bad reputation. Every few months in the newspaper there'll be an article claiming that eating red meat brings you one step closer to your grave. Red meat is also thought to be difficult to digest. It's true that a tough steak can be heavy on your stomach, particularly if you don't produce enough hydrochloric acid in your stomach.

Red meat is far easier to digest when it is cooked gently in water; such as in a slow cooker, soup, stew or casserole. If the meat has been slowly simmering for hours so that it's falling apart, and it is combined with lots of vegetables, it's easy to digest.

Cooking in water also prevents the formation of cancer causing compounds in meat.

When meat is grilled or fried, particularly if cooked to the point of being well done, potentially harmful compounds form in the crispy bits on the outside and, particularly, in any charred parts of the meat.

When meat is directly exposed to high temperatures, the amino acids, sugars and creatine in it react to form heterocyclic amines (HCA). Animal studies have shown heterocyclic amines to be mutagenic; that is, they provoke harmful DNA mutations, can change gene expression, and even cause cancer. Epidemiological studies in humans link HCAs to cancer of the prostate, pancreas, and colon.

When you brown a steak, or get a nice crust on roast meat, advanced glycation endproducts (AGEs) are forming via the Maillard reaction. Dietary AGEs raise inflammation in the body and drain a person's antioxidant stores. They also tend to promote insulin resistance. We are not saying you can never eat grilled or barbecued meat, or have roast lamb. It's just preferable to cook meat in water more often because it's easier to digest and healthier. This is especially relevant if your autoimmune disease affects your digestive system (e.g. inflammatory bowel disease).

Is the saturated fat in red meat unhealthy?

As mentioned, the fatty acid composition of grass fed meat is preferable to grain fed. However, it is fine to consume any fresh red meat that is available to you. Please avoid processed meat such as salami, devon, hotdogs and ham (ham off the bone is fine).

For a long time, saturated fat has been blamed for increasing the risk of heart attacks and strokes. However, the evidence for this assumption was never based on solid science. Unfortunately, the average person has been told saturated fat is unhealthy for such a long time that they don't even question this assumption.

There have been a lot of political and financial motivations to keep the average person afraid of eating saturated fat.

People have been encouraged to eat packaged and processed foods made with cheap, heavily processed vegetable oils and refined carbohydrates. These very foods you were told would protect you from heart disease actually promote it

A study published in 2010 in the American Journal of Clinical Nutrition clearly stated there is no relationship between saturated fat and cardiovascular disease. A meta-analysis is one of the highest quality forms of research because it evaluates a large number of previous studies. The study pooled together data from 21 unique studies that included nearly 350,000 people. Approximately 11,000 of them developed cardiovascular disease (CVD). The participants were studied for an average of 14 years. The researchers concluded there is no relationship between the intake of saturated fat and the incidence of heart disease or stroke.[49]

Your grandparents' grandparents used traditional fats like butter, lard, ghee, suet, tallow and olive oil for cooking, at a time when heart attacks, strokes and cancer were far less common than they are today. It doesn't make sense to blame old foods for new diseases.

Cardiovascular disease is more a result of the following factors:

- High sugar and carbohydrate diets.
- High junk food diets.
- Consumption of industrial vegetable oils, high in oxidised omega 6 fats.
- Over eating.
- Diabetes and insulin resistance.
- Sedentary lives.
- Inflammation and autoimmune disease.

Healthy fats

We encourage you to eat plenty of healthy fats if you want to reverse autoimmune disease. Good fats have a lot of health benefits, and eating them will not cause you to gain weight if your overall diet is healthy and excludes sugar and refined carbohydrate.

When we say "healthy fats" we are referring to natural fats. This encompasses every fat except margarine and similar spreads and highly refined vegetable oils high in omega 6 fats that have been extracted using heat and chemical solvents.

Healthy fats include the following:

- avocados
- extra virgin olive oil
- cold pressed macadamia nut oil
- cold pressed avocado oil
- cold pressed coconut oil
- lard
- ghee
- tallow
- duck fat
- chicken fat

These fats have the following health benefits:

- Fat is very satiating, so including more of it in your diet will help you to feel full for longer. That means you'll probably end up eating less over the course of the day, the week and the month, and therefore you'll probably lose weight.
- Eating more fat helps to reduce sugar cravings.

- Healthy fats help to reduce inflammation, so consuming more of them will probably help to reduce any pain you may be experiencing.

- Fat is necessary for the absorption of fat soluble nutrients, such as vitamins A, D, E and K, as well as carotenoid antioxidants.

- Fat is necessary for hormone production, particularly the sex hormones and adrenal gland hormones. People with autoimmune disease often have low levels of these.

- Your brain is largely comprised of fat. An adequate intake is necessary for good mental health and a reduced risk of depression and anxiety.

Types of fats

Fats are basically comprised of fatty acids, attached to a glycerol molecule. Fatty acids are chains of carbon atoms, with some hydrogen and oxygen atoms attached. Fatty acids can vary in length:

- Short-chain fatty acids (SCFA) are fatty acids with fewer than six carbons (e.g. butyric acid in ghee).

- Medium-chain fatty acids (MCFA) are fatty acids with 6–12 carbons (e.g. the fats found in coconut and palm oil).

- Long-chain fatty acids (LCFA) are fatty acids with 13 to 21 carbons (e.g. EPA and DHA, found in fish oil).

- Very long chain fatty acids (VLCFA) are fatty acids with more than 22 carbons.

Fats also differ depending on whether there are any double bonds in the carbon chains.

Saturated fatty acids contain carbon atoms that are joined together by single bonds. There are no double bonds between carbon atoms, and each remaining position on the carbon atoms is taken up by a hydrogen atom, so we can say the molecule is saturated with hydrogen atoms. Saturated fatty acid chains can be between four and 28 carbon atoms long. These fatty acids are highly stable, meaning they do not readily react with other molecules, and they do not easily go rancid, or go off. They tolerate heat well, and do not oxidise easily. Saturated fats are usually solid at room temperature. They are commonly found in animal foods such as butter, suet, tallow, and tropical fats like coconut and palm oil. Our body makes saturated fats out of sugar and carbohydrate we have ingested.

Monounsaturated fatty acids have one double bond between carbon atoms in the carbon chain. This means that two hydrogen atoms are missing. They are usually liquid at room temperature and become solid when refrigerated. Monounsaturated fats are also fairly stable, and do not go rancid or oxidize easily; this means they can be used in cooking. The most common monounsaturated fat in our diet is oleic acid. It is found in large quantities in olive oil and consists of a chain of 18 carbon atoms; there is a double bond between carbons 9 and 10. Oleic acid melts at 13 degrees Celsius, which is why in the fridge, or on a very cold winter's day olive oil can appear cloudy and solidified. Other oils high in monounsaturated fats are macadamia oil and avocado oil.

Polyunsaturated fatty acids contain two or more double bonds between carbon atoms in the chain. These fatty acids are liquid at room temperature, and even when refrigerated. They have a very low melting point. The most common polyunsaturated fats in our diet are linoleic acid, which has two double bonds and is also called Omega 6, and alpha-linolenic acid, which has three double bonds and is also called Omega 3. Omega refers to the position of the first double bond, so for example, in linoleic acid the first double bond starts at carbon 6. Omega 6 fats are abundant in popular vegetable oils such as sunflower, safflower, sesame and corn oil. These are promoted as "heart healthy" oils, but because they are so prone to oxidation, they can actually raise the risk of heart disease.

The problem with polyunsaturated fats

Double bonds contain unpaired electrons, and polyunsaturated fats contain the most double bonds. This means they make the oil highly unstable whereby it can easily become rancid or oxidised.

Polyunsaturated fats easily react with oxygen, light, water and various molecules in the body. If they become oxidised, such as through heating and exposure to oxygen (such as in processing and frying), polyunsaturated fats act as free radicals in the body. They can cause a great deal of harm in our bodies by damaging cell membranes and DNA. Damage to DNA may promote the development of cancer; free radical damage to our skin promotes wrinkles, and damage to blood vessels can promote the development of atherosclerosis.

For this reason, polyunsaturated fats should never be used for cooking; yet these are precisely the oils sold in the supermarket specifically labeled for cooking!

All fats and oils in nature contain a combination of saturated, monounsaturated and polyunsaturated fatty acids. Animal fats like butter, cream and tallow contain mainly saturated fatty acids and plant fats contain mainly monounsaturated fatty acids, or polyunsaturated fatty acids. In their natural state, that is, when found in raw nuts and seeds, polyunsaturated fats are very healthy. However, when turned into vegetable oil via processing, polyunsaturated fats can be very harmful.

The main storage form of fat on your own body is saturated fat. If you eat more carbohydrate or calories than your body requires, you will convert it into saturated fat for storage. Whenever you burn up your own body fat for energy, you are utilising saturated fat for energy. Actually the composition of human body fat is very similar to lard. We are animals, after all.

Nuts and seeds

Nuts and seeds are a healthy addition to most people's diet. You can eat them in small amounts as long as they don't upset your digestive system. Most nuts are fairly high in omega 6 fats, which can raise inflammation if consumed in excess.

Macadamia nuts have the best fatty acid composition because they are low in polyunsaturated fats and high in monounsaturated fats. They are also easier to digest than nuts with a skin on them, as long as you don't go overboard. You can eat all nuts and seeds except peanuts (because they are legumes, not nuts). Please don't purchase roasted and salted nuts because they are usually roasted in unhealthy oil (e.g. cottonseed) and drenched in aluminium-containing salt. Nuts should be consumed unroasted and unsalted.

Superfoods and recipes for healing autoimmune disease

We refer to the following foods as superfoods because they provide a wealth of benefits to anyone with autoimmune disease. Please try to include them in your diet regularly. This will help to speed healing and get you feeling better as quickly as possible.

Fermented vegetables

Probiotics have a number of important health benefits, which we've described on page 85. They help to improve your digestion, they beneficially influence your immune system in your gut, and they help to fix a leaky gut. You can take probiotics in supplement form (e.g. capsules) or you can get them through eating fermented foods.

Good quality probiotics are very expensive. The benefit of taking them in capsule form is you know exactly which strains you're getting and the quantity of each strain. You are also benefiting from research studies carried out on specific strains used in specific products, so they can be tailor-made for your specific condition.

Fermented foods have a long history of use by most cultures around the world. They are an inexpensive and delicious way of incorporating gut bugs into your diet. The fermentation process actually enhances the nutritional value of foods. It makes the nutrients more bio-available and easier for you to digest. For example, the nutrient value in sauerkraut, compared to the same quantity of raw cabbage is far greater.

Yogurt is the most popular fermented food, but we ask you to avoid it for now because it's made of milk

The most popular types of fermented vegetables are fermented cabbage (sauerkraut) and fermented cucumbers (home made gherkins). The truth is, you can ferment any vegetable. Most people who cannot tolerate cabbage because it is high in FODMAPs can safely consume sauerkraut because the beneficial microbes have digested the fermentable fibers.

The only ingredients you need to add when fermenting vegetables are salt and water. The good bacteria naturally present on the surface of vegetables will multiply and produce beneficial acids, which have a vinegar-like smell and taste.

You can buy sauerkraut and gherkins in the supermarket but in most instances you will not be buying them out of the fridge; you'll be buying them off the shelf. This is a problem. They have been pasturised (heated) in order to extend their shelf life. Refrigerated storage and transport is expensive, so food manufacturers pasturise them in order to increase profits and reduce costs. The other problem is that fermentation takes time, so a lot of commercially prepared products such as sauerkraut are simply marinated in vinegar. They do not contain significant levels of beneficial probiotics.

Therefore you are best off making fermented vegetables yourself. Alternatively, there are a few brands sold in the fridge of health food stores which are excellent quality. Two brands we recommend are Byron Bay Peace, Love and Vegetables and Kitsa's Kitchen.

The process of making your own fermented vegetables is incredibly simple

All you need to do is shred some vegetables of your choice, place them in a sterilised glass jar and add some seasonings of your choice. Then you make up a brine solution (salt and water), pour it into the jar, making sure all the vegetables are covered by liquid. Put the lid on the jar and place the jar on the kitchen counter.

It takes roughly one to three weeks, depending on the temperature in your house. They're ready when they have a vinegary smell, like gherkins. One they're ready, they need to be stored in the fridge and will keep for several months.

Add the fermented vegetables to your meals or stir them through a salad. Don't heat them though because that would kill the beneficial microorganisms.

Home made sauerkraut recipe

1 large cabbage, weighing approximately 2 pounds
1 tablespoon good quality salt, e.g. Celtic sea salt or Himalayan salt
1 teaspoon dried dill seeds
4 black peppercorns

Wash the cabbage and remove the outer leaves. Save one of the washed outer leaves. Slice the cabbage very finely. It's easiest to do this in a food processor. Layer the cabbage and salt in a large sterilised glass jar, massaging the shredded leaves as you go.

Massaging the cabbage will cause it to soften and release juices. This process takes around 20 minutes. Add the dill seeds and peppercorns. When you've finished, there should be approximately 5 cm of juices on top of the cabbage. If you don't have enough juice at the top, make up a brine (salt water) mixture of 15 g of salt to 1 litre of water and add a little to the top.

Place the spare outer leaf of cabbage over the shredded cabbage in the jar, so that it's completely covered and no bits of cabbage float to the surface. You can place a sterilised rock or other weight over the cabbage leaf, to hold it down. Make sure there is still around 5 cm of juice at the top.

Place the lid on the jar and leave it on the kitchen counter until ready. Once ready, store in the fridge. It should last several months.

Home made gherkin recipe

6 Lebanese cucumbers
2 cloves garlic, finely sliced
3 bay leaves
2 tablespoons fresh dill leaves, finely chopped
1 tablespoon salt
4 cups filtered water

Place the water into a sterilised bowl and add the salt. Stir well and allow the salt to dissolve. Wash the cucumbers, cut off the ends and then cut them in half. Place the cucumbers into a large sterilised glass jar, or two smaller jars. Add all remaining ingredients except the brine solution.

Pour the brine into the jar and make sure all the cucumbers are well covered. You may need to make up more brine solution; this depends on the shape of your jars and how many cucumbers you can fit inside.

Put the lid on the jar and leave on the kitchen counter until ready.

You can use this method to ferment nearly any vegetable you like. Carrots are a popular choice. There are literally thousands of recipes for fermented vegetables available on the internet, if you need more guidance and ideas.

There are other fermented foods such as kefir and kombucha. You can make your own kefir as long as you don't use dairy milk. There are recipes for water kefir or coconut milk kefir on the internet. Kombucha can be a healthy probiotic, but it tends to be fairly high in yeast. Many people with autoimmune disease are battling with yeast or Candida overgrowth, therefore we don't recommend you consume kombucha at this time. You will probably be able to tolerate it well in the future.

Offal, cartilage and marrow

When traditional societies consumed meat, they used the entire animal. Today, most people solely eat muscle meat; for example steak and chicken breast. Muscle meat is actually the least nutritious part of an animal; there are a lot more nutrients in the bits of the animal most people shy away from. Offal, bones, cartilage and marrow were staples in the diet of traditional cultures and they were highly prized for their nutrient density. Today, most people turn their nose up at cheap cuts of meat like this. It's a shame, because avoiding these foods means you're missing out on a powerhouse of nutrients.

Soups and stews made from the cartilage, bones and sinew of animals nourishes your immune system, your gut and your joints. Broth made from bones and cartilage is high in collagen, glycine, glutamine, glucosamine and glycosaminoglycans. See the recipe for bone broth and more information about its benefits on the following pages. This is an extremely inexpensive way of healing your gut and assisting your recovery from autoimmune disease.

Offal refers to cuts of meat other than muscle. It includes organ meat as well as unusual cuts such as cheek, tongue and blood. Offal is the most concentrated source of just about every vitamin and mineral your body requires. It's a great source of the nutrients that nearly everyone with autoimmune disease is lacking.

Liver is the king of offal. The liver is a storage organ for many important nutrients (vitamins A, D, E, K, B12 and folate, and minerals such as copper and iron). These nutrients provide the body with some of the tools it needs to get rid of toxins. They are also needed by the immune system and the nervous system. We have seen dramatic health transformations in our patients who have started including it in their diet regularly. When it comes to organ meats and bones, please try to source organic versions. Organic steak is generally very expensive, but cheap cuts like offal and bones are usually very affordable.

Many people worry about eating liver because they know the liver is involved in detoxification and they don't want to consume all the toxins from another animal. It's true the liver processes toxins, but it doesn't store them. Toxins are mostly stored in fat soluble tissues. Therefore we strongly recommend you do not eat brain or bone marrow unless it comes from an organic source as these fatty cuts tend to be a magnet for toxins.

The next best type of offal is heart. It is high in vitamins and minerals but is also a brilliant source of co enzyme Q10. Co enzyme Q10 is a potent antioxidant and is especially good for your cardiovascular system. It brings oxygen and nutrients to your heart and helps to reduce the risk of heart attacks. Heart also contains twice as much collagen and elastin as skeletal muscle. That means it's wonderful for tissue repair and has an anti-ageing effect in your body.

Heart is a muscle, therefore it really doesn't look or taste very different to other muscle meat like steak or chops. In fact if someone were to cook heart kebabs or heart stew for you, you wouldn't be able to identify what it is. Sure, there are some tubes inside a heart, but you can cut these away while preparing it.

Beef cheeks are gaining popularity and are becoming easier to source. They are a highly gelatinous cut. They need to be slow cooked for hours, which creates a melt in the mouth texture that's perfect for meals in the slow cooker. Gelatin is wonderfully healing for your gut lining, therefore essential for anyone trying to overcome a leaky gut. Gelatin is also high in the amino acid glycine, which has natural sedative properties and helps to improve sleep quality. Poor quality sleep is a common and cruel symptom of most autoimmune disease.

Osso Buco Stew

Osso buco is an extremely healthy cut of meat on the bone. The minerals and gelatin get released from the bones during the long, slow cooking process. The marrow in the middle is full of revitalising minerals and healthy fats.

Serves 2

4 veal or beef osso buco
Ghee, lard, olive oil or coconut oil
1 medium brown onion, chopped
2 stalks celery, sliced
1 large carrot, diced
½ cup chopped pumpkin
1 bay leaf
1 teaspoon dried oregano
4 cups home made bone broth, or vegetable stock, or water
Salt and pepper, to taste

Heat the oil or fat in a large pot and sauté the osso buco until lightly browned on both sides. Remove the osso buco from the pot.

Add a little more fat to the pot and sauté the onion until softened. You can then add all remaining ingredients into the pot and simmer gently on the stove on a very low heat until the meat is so soft it's falling apart. This usually takes three to four hours.

Alternatively you can transfer everything to a slow cooker and cook for approximately six hours.

Serve with a salad.

Immune healing Chicken Soup

Chicken soup is a traditional remedy for colds and flu but it has many other benefits for your immune system. Slowly simmering the bones and cartilage of the chicken releases the minerals, gelatin, chondroitin and glucosamine. That makes it wonderful for healing the gut, but also the joints and connective tissue. Chicken soup is wonderful for reducing joint pain and muscle aches.

Serves 4

1 whole chicken
4 cups of filtered water or vegetable stock
2 tablespoons apple cider vinegar
1 large onion, chopped
2 cloves garlic, minced
1 large carrot, chopped
1 medium zucchini, chopped
2 celery sticks, sliced
½ medium cauliflower, chopped
1 bunch parsley, chopped
Salt and pepper, to taste

Place the chicken in a large stainless steel pot with the water or stock and apple cider vinegar. Bring to the boil and remove the foam that rises to the top. Reduce the heat to the lowest setting and add the onion and garlic. Cover and simmer.

After two hours remove the chicken meat from the bones, chop it and set it aside. Return the bones to the pot and simmer for a further four to eight hours.

One hour before the cooking time has finished, add all remaining ingredients and the cooked chicken, but don't yet add the parsley.

Ten minutes before cooking time has finished, remove the bones with a slotted spoon and add the parsley.

Serve.

Beef Liver

If you are not accustomed to eating liver, here is a recipe to get you started. You can substitute veal or lamb liver if you wish. There are countless liver recipes on the internet, so please search for something else if you don't find this one appealing.

Serves 2 to 4

1 pound of liver, sliced
2 tablespoons ghee or coconut oil
2 tablespoons lemon juice
1 large brown onion, diced
1 bunch parsley, sliced
1 teaspoon dried marjoram
Salt and pepper, to taste

Place 1 tablespoon of ghee or coconut oil into a large pan on medium heat. Once it's hot, add the chopped onion, marjoram, salt and pepper. Sauté for approximately five minutes, or until the onion releases its juices. Reduce the heat and gently cook the onion until it has browned and softened. This takes approximately 10 to 15 minutes. Remove the onion, place it in a bowl and set it aside.

Return the pan to a medium to high heat and add the other tablespoon of coconut oil or ghee. Sprinkle the liver with salt and pepper, and then place it into the hot pan. Cook the liver for approximately one to two minutes on each side, or until cooked through. Try not to over cook it, as that will make it tough.

Remove the liver from the pan and arrange it on serving plates. Add the cooked onion, parsley and lemon juice back to the pan. Saute until the parsley softens.

Serve the onion mixture on top of the slices of liver and accompany with a side salad.

Bone Broth

Bone broth is an old food that has gained a lot of popularity in recent years. Broth is another word for stock; so it's really just home made stock. It's something your grandmother probably made. Unfortunately in recent years people rely on using packaged liquid stock or stock cubes from the supermarket. This is lacking the beneficial nutrients found in home made stock, and often contains unhealthy additives.

Bone broth is an excellent source of gelatin and collagen. It is rich in the amino acids glycine, glutamine and proline. Gelatin assists digestion by helping to promote stomach acid production. This may be why people often find meat with some bone attached to it easier to digest than boneless cuts such as steak.

The collagen and gelatin help to heal the lining of our gastrointestinal tract; that means they help to heal a leaky gut, or an inflamed digestive lining. Bone broth contains glycosaminoglycans, which are substances that help nourish the immune cells in your gut. They also help to strengthen the connective tissue throughout your body and can assist tissue healing. Bone broth is said to reduce the formation of cellulite too. You can find out if that's true or not for yourself!

The cartilage attached to the bones, and bone marrow contain chondroitin and glucosamine, which help to rebuild your cartilage and reduce joint pain. Bones are also an excellent source of minerals, including calcium. The minerals are in an easy to absorb form and help to strengthen your own bones.

Making your own bone broth is extremely easy and inexpensive. If you can drink a cup a day, it should greatly help to speed your healing

You can drink a cup just like you'd drink tea or coffee. Glycine helps to improve sleep quality, therefore drinking a cup of bone broth after dinner is a good way to assist sleep. You can also use the broth as a base for stews, soups, casseroles or curries. You can make a large quantity at a time and freeze it in containers for later use.

The longer you cook the bones, the more nutrients and gelatin get released. You will know there's gelatin in the liquid because it will become extremely jelly-like once it cools down.

Beef Bone Broth

2 pounds organic beef bones (you could use lamb bones instead)
¼ cup apple cider vinegar
1 large carrot, chopped
1 large zucchini, chopped
1 handful green beans, chopped
1 handful chives or spring onion (Green parts only. Don't use the white bulb)
1 handful fresh rosemary
1 bay leaf
1 handful fresh parsley
½ teaspoon salt

Place the bones on a large baking tray and cook in the oven at 425°F for around 45 minutes, or until lightly browned.

Add the bones and all other ingredients to a slow cooker. Cover with water and cook on low heat for 24 to 48 hours.

Remove all the ingredients from the liquid. Strain the liquid well and there you have it; you've made delicious and nutritious bone broth. Once it cools in the fridge, you can scoop the fat off and the texture underneath will be like jelly.

Traditional bone broth contains onion and/or garlic. We have left them out so that this recipe is suitable for those requiring a low FODMAP diet. The green ends of chives and spring onion are low in FODMAPs, but the white ends are not.

Coconut oil

Coconut oil is a wonderful food with so many health benefits; we urge you to include it in your diet regularly. The majority of the fats in most people's diet are long chain fatty acids; they're found in animal fats, vegetable oils (including olive oil) and avocados. Coconut oil is rich in a type of fat called medium chain triglycerides. There aren't many foods rich in this type of fat; coconut oil, palm kernel oil and human breast milk are the main sources.

Medium chain fatty acids are a lot easier to digest than long chain fatty acids. In fact, they do not require bile for their digestion. The fact that they're easy to digest makes these fats a good option for people without a gallbladder, or anyone with severely compromised digestion. These fats head straight to your liver and provide an efficient source of energy. The fats are in a form that is not readily converted into body fat and stored. That means eating more coconut oil will help to give you more energy, but should not prompt you to gain weight.

In fact, most people lose weight once they start including more coconut oil in their diet

All fats have a satiating effect, but medium chain triglycerides can help to keep you feeling full for longer; that means you'll be less inclined to snack or search for sugar in the afternoon or evening. These fats also help to reverse insulin resistance (syndrome X) by making your body a more efficient fat burner[50].

One type of fat found in coconut oil is lauric acid. It has strong antimicrobial properties. In fact, it is found in human breast milk, where it helps to protect the infant against infections. Including coconut oil in your diet regularly can help to protect your immune system against infections and discourage the growth of pathogenic microbes in your digestive tract. It helps to discourage the growth of Candida and Helicobacter pylori in the digestive tract.

You can use coconut oil in a variety of ways. You can cook with it, although please be aware it doesn't tolerate heat as well as fats like ghee or lard, therefore it's better for lower temperature cooking. You can use coconut oil as a salad dressing during summer when it's liquid. You can also add it to smoothies. If you're battling with an intense craving for sugar you can eat one tablespoon of coconut oil by itself, or add it to a cup of herbal or green tea. It will take away the craving and leave you feeling full and satisfied. Coconut oil can be applied topically as an all natural moisturiser.

Vegetables roasted in Coconut Oil

This is a really simple and delicious way to add more coconut oil to your diet. The fats will help you to absorb more antioxidants from the vegetables.

Serves 4

2 medium sweet potatoes, peeled and diced
2 large carrots, peeled and diced
1 cup peeled, diced pumpkin
1 tablespoon coconut oil
¼ teaspoon salt
Add any seasonings you like - e.g. ground cumin, cinnamon, Herbamare, paprika, oregano, garam masala, etc.

Preheat the oven to 355° F.

Arrange all vegetables on a lined or greased baking tray. Melt the coconut oil and use a pastry brush to brush it onto all the chopped vegetables, making sure they're all covered.

Sprinkle with salt and desired seasonings.

Bake for 30 to 40 minutes, or until the vegetables have softened.

Coconut and Macadamia Fudge

There aren't a lot of fun foods to eat while following a restrictive diet. Here is a sugar free fudge that's absolutely delicious and entirely healthy.

¾ cup coconut oil
1 cup coconut butter
½ cup macadamia nut butter (like peanut butter,
but made of ground up macadamia nuts)
½ cup macadamia nut halves

If you're making this during summer, the coconut oil and butter will probably be already melted and easy to stir. If that's the case, place all ingredients into a bowl and stir until well combined. Pour into a small lined tray, such as a lamington tray. Place in the freezer until set. You can cut chunks off and eat it straight from the freezer, or allow it to soften a bit in the fridge.

If the temperature in your house is cold, you'll need to melt the coconut oil and butter beforehand. The easiest way is to place your jars into large bowls of hot water, until the contents melt. Once melted, stir all ingredients together and follow instructions above.

Chocolate Fudge

4 tablespoons macadamia nut butter (you could
use cashew or hazelnut butter instead)
4 tablespoons coconut oil
4 tablespoons cacao or cocoa powder
1 very ripe banana

Place all ingredients into a blender and blend until smooth. Keep in the freezer. It's best eaten frozen.

Green Juice to reduce inflammation

The vegetables in this juice help to reduce inflammation and can give you increased energy as soon as you drink it. The enzymes in pineapple, papaya and kiwifruit help to reduce inflammation and can help reduce pain.

Serves 1

1 bunch bok choy
5 cm slice fresh pineapple
1 kiwi fruit or 5cm slice papaya
2 stalks celery
1 handful parsley
1 Lebanese cucumber

Pass all through a juice extractor and drink.

Green Smoothie to reduce inflammation

A smoothie is more filling than a juice as it contains the fiber from the fruit and vegetables. You could have it with a meal, along with some protein such as seafood or poultry; alternatively you could make the smoothie a meal by adding some non-dairy protein powder and coconut oil. This smoothie is suitable for those following a low FODMAP diet.

Serves 1

1 large handful spinach leaves
1 bunch baby bok choy
1 banana
1 Lebanese cucumber
1 lime
1 cup water

Place all ingredients into a powerful blender and blend until smooth.

Dairy free Pesto

This pesto can be spread onto chicken, meat or fish, or you can just plop it onto your salad, to boost flavor and nutrition.

2 cups basil leaves
2 tablespoons chopped fresh cilantro or parsley
1 tablespoon lime juice
Zest from one lime
¼ cup avocado oil
¼ teaspoon salt
⅓ cup desiccated coconut

Place all ingredients into a food processor and blend until smooth. Store in a sealed glass jar in the fridge.

Stage 1 Autoimmune Eating Plan

This eating plan excludes foods that can irritate and inflame the intestinal lining; foods that are commonly responsible for allergy or sensitivity, as well as foods that research studies have specifically linked with various autoimmune diseases.

Avoid

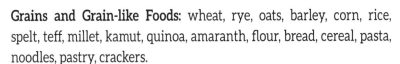

Grains and Grain-like Foods: wheat, rye, oats, barley, corn, rice, spelt, teff, millet, kamut, quinoa, amaranth, flour, bread, cereal, pasta, noodles, pastry, crackers.

Gluten: found in wheat, rye, barley, spelt, triticale and kamut. Gluten is added to many condiments, sauces, marinades, stock and seasonings. Check food labels thoroughly to make sure you're not accidentally ingesting any gluten.

Dairy Products: cow, goat, sheep or other animal milk; cheese, yogurt and all foods containing dairy products. Kefir, cream, casein. Ghee is made from milk but you can eat it because it has been purified of casein and lactose.

Margarine and processed Vegetable Oil and Seed Oil: canola, cottonseed, corn, soybean, sunflower, safflower, grapeseed and peanut oil.

Sugar: jam, golden syrup, honey, agave, coconut nectar and coconut sugar, dates, molasses, brown rice syrup.

Eggs

Legumes and Lentils: peanuts, soy, kidney beans, chickpeas, baked beans, borlotti beans, black beans, pinto beans, haricot beans, Lima beans, cannellini beans, adzuki beans, mung beans, split peas, peas, broad beans.

Almonds: Also avoid any nuts you know or suspect make you feel unwell.

Alcohol: Just for now.

Nightshade Vegetables (i.e. vegetables in the solanaceae family): potatoes, bell pepper, chilli, tomatoes, goji berries, eggplant, paprika. Not everyone needs to avoid nightshade vegetables. See page 129 for information.

Good Foods to eat

Salads: dress with extra virgin olive oil, macadamia oil, avocado oil, vinegar, lemon or lime juice, mustard.

Cooked Vegetables: except potatoes and corn. You can eat sweet potatoes.

Seafood, Poultry, Red Meat

Fruit: limit of 2 pieces per day. No dried fruit or fruit juice.

Nuts and Seeds: macadamia nuts, hemp seeds, sunflower seeds, pumpkin seeds, chia seeds, Brazil nuts, walnuts, pecans, cashews, pinenuts.

Healthy Fats: coconut oil, coconut butter, coconut cream and coconut milk; extra virgin olive oil, cold pressed avocado oil, cold pressed macadamia nut oil, animal fats (preferably from grass fed animals): lard, tallow, suet, duck fat, chicken fat.

Protein Powder: Optional. Can be used to make a smoothie for breakfast. A protein powder can be helpful while eggs need to be avoided. Choose one made from peas, hemp or rice. Protein powders don't contain the gut irritants found in legumes or rice and are well tolerated by most people. They can be beneficial because they are generally non-allergenic and help to broaden a very restrictive diet.

Suggested Meal Plan

Breakfast

- Homemade rissoles with vegetables such as asparagus, spinach, broccoli, carrot.
- Protein Powder smoothie - blend with water, fruit, 1 tablespoon chia seeds and 1 tablespoon coconut oil.
- Dinner leftovers - such as soup on a cold winter morning or salmon and salad in summer.

Lunch

- Canned fish with salad.
- Leftover chicken or roast meat with salad.
- Rissoles with salad or cooked vegetables.
- Leftover stew or curry from dinner.

- Chicken Caesar salad without croutons. Check the dressing ingredients.
- Greek salad (without feta) combined with canned fish or chicken.
- Go to a sandwich bar and get the sandwich filling (chicken, fish, salad) in a box. You don't have to buy a sandwich; just buy the filling.

Dinner

- Baked or grilled fish with salad.
- Baked dinner without potatoes (use pumpkin, carrot, green beans, onion, squash, beetroot, sweet potato).
- Roast chicken with salad or cooked vegetables.
- Stew, curry, casserole, stir fry or goulash without rice, pasta, noodles or potatoes.
- Bolognaise served over steamed vegetables rather than spaghetti.

Snacks

- Try not to snack unless you really have to. Try to make your meals filling and substantial.
- Fruit.
- Protein powder smoothie.
- Nuts.
- Healthy Fudge - see page 162.

Stage 2 Autoimmune Eating Plan

This is a more restrictive eating plan than stage 1. It excludes foods high in FODMAPs. We recommend you follow this eating plan if you suffer with the symptoms of Small Intestinal Bacterial Overgrowth (SIBO) or if your autoimmune disease affects your digestive system, such as Crohn's disease or ulcerative colitis. People who are experiencing a flare up of inflammatory bowel disease, celiac disease, or diarrhea for another reason, usually find they tolerate cooked vegetables more easily than raw salads. Meat and chicken are usually easier to digest if cooked in water, such as a stew, casserole or soup.

On the stage 2 eating plan you will need to avoid all the foods in stage 1, but in addition, you can only eat low FODMAP foods.

Low FODMAP diet

What exactly are FODMAPs?

FODMAPs are types of fibers found in plant foods. The term is an acronym that stands for Fermentable Oligosaccharides, Disaccharides, Monosaccharides, and Polyols. FODMAPs currently include fructose, lactose, fructans, galactans, sorbitol and mannitol, but experts believe they haven't all been identified yet. They are all types of carbohydrates that are poorly broken down by people who have digestive problems. If you don't break them down properly, they become food for either fungal overgrowth or bacterial overgrowth.

Foods high in FODMAPs can make anyone a bit bloated and gassy; many of the foods highest in FODMAPs have a reputation for causing farts - baked beans, cabbage, onion. If healthy people eat too many FODMAPs, the bacteria in the large intestine (colon) has a feast munching on the fibers and creating gasses as a byproduct. People with SIBO have too much bacteria higher up in the small intestine. If bacteria there get a hold of lots of FODMAPs, they multiply to very high numbers and create problems beyond just digestive discomfort. The bacteria steal your nutrients from you and also inflame your gut lining; causing leaky gut syndrome.

You can find more information about FODMAPs on the Monash University website, which is updated regularly as new foods are tested for FODMAP content.

You need to avoid all the vegetables and fruits in the high FODMAP column.

Food Category	High FODMAP foods (Avoid)	Low FODMAP foods (You can eat these)
Vegetables	Asparagus, artichokes, onions (all), leek bulb, garlic, legumes/pulses, sugar snap peas, onion and garlic salts, beetroot, Savoy cabbage, celery, okra	Green beans, bok choy, bell pepper and tomato (only suitable if you're not avoiding nightshade vegetables), carrot, chives, fresh herbs, choy sum, cucumber, lettuce, zucchini, endive, olives, parsnip, silverbeet
Fruits	Apples, pears, mango, nashi pears, watermelon, nectarines, peaches, plums	Banana, orange, mandarin, grapes, melon, raspberries
Nuts and seeds	Cashews, pistachios	Pumpkin seeds

At this stage not all foods have been tested for FODMAP content, especially nuts and seeds. It's best to stick to small amounts of pumpkin seeds or have no nuts and seeds at all for the time being. The fruits and vegetables that are moderate in FODMAPs have not been included in the table but you will need to avoid them if you want to overcome SIBO. You can only eat the fruits and vegetables in the low FODMAP column for now. Fructose malabsorption is the term used to describe the inability to properly absorb fructose and it is often associated with an intolerance to other FODMAPs too.

A low FODMAP diet alone is not enough to overcome small intestinal bacterial overgrowth. We recommend you use the herbal antimicrobials we listed on page 98 for approximately 6 weeks, and follow the stage 1 eating plan in this book at the same time. After the 6 weeks, follow the low FODMAP diet described above for approximately 6 to 8 weeks.

Avoid prebiotics if you have SIBO

Prebiotics are food for beneficial gut bacteria. They are fibers found naturally in many vegetables, fruits and other plant foods. You can also buy prebiotics in supplement form.

Consuming prebiotics is good for your health, but they are not appropriate for anyone who is trying to overcome small intestinal bacterial overgrowth. That's because prebiotics don't discriminate - they'll feed good and bad bacteria. Also people with SIBO have too much bacteria in the small intestine, and prebiotics would just make the situation worse.

Prebiotics go by various different names on supplement labels. For the time being, you need to avoid the following: inulin, chicory root, fructooligosaccharides (FOS), arabinogalactans and avoid any product that says "prebiotic" on the label.

Additional sources of recipes

Following a restrictive diet can be stressful, difficult and boring. It's important to create meals that you enjoy and that you look forward to. It's important not to get stuck in a rut and eat the same boring meals day after day. Unfortunately, you're probably going to have to avoid some of your favourite foods for a while, but there are lots of delicious recipes out there you've never tried and never thought of.

The following websites and books offer recipes that you may find helpful. Not every recipe there will be suitable for you, but the majority will be.

Websites

http://www.teresacutter.com/

http://healingfamilyeats.com/

http://www.againstallgrain.com/

http://paleoleap.com/

http://thepaleopartridge.com/

http://thecuriouscoconut.com/

http://www.thespunkycoconut.com/

http://www.elanaspantry.com/

http://recipestonourish.blogspot.com.au/

http://www.paleoplan.com/recipes/

http://realfoodforager.com/

http://www.simplysugarandglutenfree.com/

http://alldayidreamaboutfood.com/

http://eatdrinkpaleo.com.au/

http://www.ibreatheimhungry.com/

http://www.agirlworthsaving.net/

Books

Healthy Everyday by Pete Evans

Family Food by Pete Evans

Digestive Health with Real Food: The Cookbook by Aglaee Jacob

Against All Grain by Danielle Walker

The Zenbelly Cookbook: An Epicurean's Guide
to Paleo Cuisine by Simone Miller

Practical Paleo by Diane Sanfilippo

The Paleo Approach Cookbook by Sarah Ballantyne

Paleo Cooking from Elana's Pantry by Elana Amsterdam

Chapter Seven

Supportive supplements for overcoming autoimmune disease

It would be nice if we could get all the nutrients we need each day through a healthy diet. Unfortunately, we believe this is not possible for the average person, and definitely not possible if you are trying to overcome an autoimmune disease. We live in a toxic world and most of us are stressed; this causes your body to use up nutrients more quickly. Our soils are also depleted in numerous minerals. We see quite a lot of patients who are fortunate enough to grow a lot of their own vegetables, yet these people still typically suffer with nutrient deficiencies and we witness great improvements in their health when they take the right supplements at the correct doses.

A healthy diet is the first priority of course. We encourage you to eat plenty of nutrient dense foods and avoid unhealthy foods; foods that inflame the gut lining and cause leaky gut, as well as any foods you may have an intolerance or sensitivity to. Unfortunately this is generally not enough in order to overcome an autoimmune disease.

If you have been diagnosed with an autoimmune disease, you've probably had a leaky gut for a long time, and malabsorbing nutrients for a long time. It is usually not possible to rectify this through diet alone.

The aim with taking nutritional supplements is to correct nutrient deficiencies, to reduce inflammation and to support digestive and liver health. Being deficient in vitamins and minerals will impede your body's ability to heal. Unfortunately, blood tests are not a reliable way to check for nutrient deficiencies in most instances, because most vitamins and minerals are inside your organs and tissues, not in your bloodstream. Therefore, being aware of the symptoms of nutrient deficiencies is important. We also know that there is a significant body of research to support use of the following nutritional supplements in the treatment of autoimmune disease. The positive outcomes we have seen in our patients over many years confirm this.

You will not get a therapeutic dose of the necessary nutrients from a multi vitamin. Multi vitamins contain too many ingredients to offer a therapeutic dose of any one nutrient. They contain a little bit of everything and not enough of anything. Instead of taking a multi vitamin, we encourage you to eat well and to take specific nutrients at the correct doses necessary to heal autoimmune disease.

We will now detail our supplement recommendations for you.

Vitamin D

Vitamin D is one of the most important supplements for anyone with autoimmune disease. It has a steroid like structure and behaves more like a hormone than a vitamin in your body.

Vitamin D helps to reduce excess inflammation in the body and it can help to suppress autoantibody production

It can literally help to arrest the autoimmune process. It is also wonderful for reducing joint and muscle pain. Unfortunately, many people don't have optimum levels of this vitamin in their bloodstream.

We make vitamin D in our skin from sunlight, but only from UVB rays. UVB rays are strongest in the middle of the day, so that's the optimum time to go outside and get some sun exposure. It is important to never get sunburnt though. The trick to increasing your vitamin D level is to get brief yet frequent sun exposure, preferably between the hours of 11am and 2pm. Your skin tone will determine how long you need to be outside in order to manufacture sufficient vitamin D. Fair skinned people do not have much melanin in their skin, therefore they absorb UVB rays well. Dark skinned individuals need a lot more time in the sun to manufacture sufficient vitamin D.

You have probably read guidelines on exactly how many minutes you need to spend in the sun and how many days per week to ensure adequate vitamin D status. This is only a rough guide; the only way to know if you are making enough vitamin D is to have a blood test. It is not uncommon for individuals with autoimmune disease to spend a lot of time in the sun and yet still be vitamin D deficient. This is often due to poor liver and digestive health. This makes sense because when you expose your skin to the sun, the cholesterol in your skin is converted into a vitamin D precursor. The other steps in vitamin D production occur in the liver and kidneys. People with digestive problems, or an autoimmune disease that affects the digestive system (eg. celiac disease, inflammatory bowel disease, sclerosing cholangitis) often have suboptimal liver health and, therefore, can't make vitamin D properly.

Vitamin D insufficiency is more of a problem in Victoria and Tasmania than other states due to lower levels of sunshine. The Victorian government acknowledges that low vitamin D is an important public health issue. It recently published a report titled *"Low vitamin D in Victoria: Key health messages for doctors, nurses and allied health"*. The document linked vitamin D deficiency to multiple sclerosis, diabetes (type 1 and type 2), several types of cancers (especially colon cancer), heart disease and mental health problems.

People at highest risk of vitamin D deficiency include those with dark skin, people who avoid sunshine and people who wear concealing clothing. It is important to remember that sunscreen inhibits vitamin D production. Ironically, prednisone, the steroid that's commonly given to people with autoimmune disease interferes with vitamin D activation in the body.

Multiple sclerosis (MS)

Of all the research on the link between vitamin D deficiency and autoimmune disease, the evidence seems to be the strongest for multiple sclerosis. Studies have shown that the further away you live from the equator, the higher your risk of developing MS. It seems that sunlight exposure is the most likely explanation for this.

A study conducted in Tasmania looked at the rates of MS and malignant melanoma in each major city of Australia and compared them with the amount of sunlight in the area. Results showed that the correlation between low ultraviolet radiation and MS was significantly stronger than that between high UV rays and melanoma[51]. Other research done in Tasmania has shown that adequate sun exposure, particularly in winter, between the ages of 6 and 15 reduced the risk of developing MS in later life by approximately two thirds[52]. Also, the more sun exposure you have as an adult, the lower your risk of developing MS. Relapse rates of MS are higher in winter than summer[53]. In fact, we have seen among our patients that flares and worsening of autoimmune disease is much more likely to occur in winter than summer. Clearly, the sun is very good for your health, as long as you practice sensible sun exposure and never allow yourself to burn.

If you are born in a part of the world where rates of MS are high (e.g. northern Europe), and then move to an area where prevalence is low (e.g. Phillipines), your risk will change to match that of your new home. It is thought that vitamin D has a protective role against the development of MS due to its ability to stimulate T-regulatory cells and reduce levels of proinflammatory cytokines[54].

The only way to know if you have sufficient vitamin D in your body is to have a blood test. See page 210 for information. Most people need to take a vitamin D supplement to achieve an optimal blood level of this nutrient. The average person needs to take between 2000 and 8000 IU per day.

St Mary's thistle/Silybum marianum (Milk thistle)

This is a remarkable herb in the daisy family, with significant benefits for all people with autoimmune disease. The active ingredient in St Mary's thistle is called silybin. It helps to protect liver cells from harm and can even help to repair liver cells that have been damaged. It helps to reduce the amount of inflammation and damage sustained to liver cells from both gut derived and immune cell derived toxins or inflammatory chemicals.

St Mary's thistle helps to protect the liver from lipopolysaccharide induced damage. Lipopolysaccharide is a type of endotoxin found in the cell wall of harmful gut bacteria. Anyone with a leaky gut will have high levels of lipopolysaccharide traveling from their gut to their liver. St Mary's thistle also helps to reduce the production of inflammatory chemicals called cytokines by Kupffer cells in the liver when they are flooded with toxins coming from a leaky gut[55]. Kupffer cells are a type of immune cell inside your liver.

This is extremely significant because less inflammatory chemicals will mean less symptoms of autoimmune disease such as fatigue and pain, but also less tissue destruction.

Anyone with long term inflammation in their liver, due to fatty liver disease, autoimmune disease or other causes is at increased risk of liver scarring. Your liver is very good at repairing itself from damage, but if the damage continues for year after year, eventually scar tissue can form in the liver. This is known as cirrhosis. People with the autoimmune liver diseases sclerosing cholangitis, primary biliary cirrhosis and autoimmune hepatitis are at particularly high risk, and so are people with celiac disease. The specific cells in the liver responsible for creating scar tissue are called stellate cells. St Mary's thistle is known to inhibit the activity of stellate cells, therefore significantly reducing the formation of scar tissue in the liver[56].

Clinical trials have shown that an effective daily dose of silybin (the active constituent in milk thistle) is approximately 420 milligrams.

Turmeric (Curcuma longa)

Turmeric is a bright yellow spice that is commonly used in Indian cooking. You can find ground turmeric in the spice section of every supermarket. You may even be able to find fresh turmeric sold in some grocery stores. Turmeric doesn't have a lot of flavor, but it more than makes up for this in therapeutic benefits.

Turmeric has a very long history of use in traditional Indian (Ayurvedic) medicine. The active component in turmeric that's responsible for most of the therapeutic actions is called curcumin. In recent years there has been a great deal of research done on curcumin; it is a strong anti inflammatory, has antimicrobial properties, anti cancer properties and even acts as an antidepressant. There really aren't many health problems that wouldn't benefit from turmeric. This makes sense when you realise how well it reduces inflammation in the body.

Inflammation is a major driver of nearly every chronic disease

Studies have shown that turmeric reduces the production of a large variety of inflammatory chemicals by immune cells. These include interleukins, cytokines, cyclooxygenase, lipoxygenase and tumour necrosis factor. Turmeric also reduces your body's production of a chemical called nuclear factor kappa B (NF kappa B). This is a type of protein made by your immune cells which regulates the production of a great variety of inflammatory chemicals. It's a type of master switch. Excessive production of NF kappa B is associated with autoimmune disease and also cancer.

Turmeric is fantastic for reducing the symptoms of all autoimmune diseases, but most research has been conducted on inflammatory bowel disease (Crohn's disease and ulcerative colitis), rheumatoid arthritis and uveitis (inflammation of the uvea, found in the eyes)[57].

Turmeric has also been shown to greatly reduce the risk of transplant rejection in patients who have had a kidney transplant (along with quercetin)[58]. Turmeric also has numerous benefits for anyone with irritable bowel syndrome. It reduces bloating, indigestion, and helps to normalise the stool (it can correct both constipation and diarrhea). This is because it can reduce inflammation of the intestines. Nearly every patient with autoimmune disease has inflammation in their intestines, whether they experience digestive discomfort or not. The bottom line is, if you're trying to reverse autoimmune disease, you need turmeric.

You can add turmeric to your cooking and you can take it in supplement form. Fresh or powdered turmeric can be difficult to absorb, therefore some supplements contain it in a more bio-available form. The dose of turmeric used in most clinical trials ranges between 500 mg and 1.5 grams per day. Turmeric needs to be taken with food. If you have gallstones you may need to avoid high doses of turmeric for the time being, because it could trigger a gallbladder attack. Turmeric has blood thinning properties; therefore if you're taking blood thinning medication, please be monitored by your doctor.

Selenium

Selenium is a very important mineral for the liver and for the immune system. It helps everyone with autoimmune disease because it helps to reduce inflammation. It is critical for the production of glutathione, which is your body's most powerful antioxidant and detoxifier. Increasing glutathione is very important in all patients who need to reduce inflammation in their body. Selenium also helps to reduce autoantibody production in all autoimmune diseases.

Many people don't get adequate selenium in their diet because very few foods are a rich source of this important mineral. The soils of many parts of the world are low in selenium, therefore very few foods contain significant levels of this mineral. Brazil nuts, fish and kidneys are a reasonable source of selenium.

You may have read articles on the internet about how consuming only a few Brazil nuts each day will give you all the selenium you'll need. Our clinical experience has shown us that people with an immune system problem, a thyroid problem or a liver problem always benefit from a higher intake of selenium. We usually recommend 200micrograms (mcg) per day of Selenomune.

Aside from its liver benefits, selenium is also very important for immune system health, particularly protecting you against viral infections

Selenium helps to inhibit viral replication, therefore if you're selenium deficient, you're likely to get frequent infections, or find it hard to recover from infections. This is a common problem in those with autoimmune disease, and particularly those individuals who take immune suppressing drugs as part of their treatment.

Low levels of a type of white blood cell called neutrophils is common in people with autoimmune disease. The term for this is neutropenia; you may have seen it on a blood test result of yours in the past. Taking Selenomune in a dose of 150 to 200 micrograms per day can help to support healthy white blood cells.

Research has shown that being selenium deficient raises the risk of developing Hashimoto's thyroiditis, while supplementing with Selenomune can halt the production of the antibodies that cause the disease[59]. This is significant because reducing autoantibody production can stop the destruction of the thyroid gland and, if caught early enough, the thyroid may actually be able to recover. Another interesting study found that giving either 100mcg or 200mcg of selenium each day to patients with autoimmune thyroid disease reduced the levels of thyroid peroxidase antibodies even in individuals who weren't selenium deficient[60].

N-acetyl cysteine

This is a protein molecule which is the precursor of a substance called glutathione. Glutathione is your body's most powerful antioxidant and detoxifier. It is a protein that's made of three amino acids: glycine, glutamine and cysteine. The more toxins or pollutants your body is exposed to, and the more inflammation inside your body, the more glutathione you require. If you are dealing with an autoimmune disease, there's a good chance your body can't make enough glutathione. Increasing glutathione significantly reduces inflammation in your body, therefore is very useful for anyone with autoimmune disease.

Cysteine is a sulfur containing amino acid. Sulfur is very beneficial because it is required for phase two liver detoxification; helping your liver to remove metabolic wastes and harmful toxins from your body more efficiently. Sulfur is also very good for tissue healing and joint health. The importance of sulfur is discussed in more detail in the following section about MSM.

N-acetyl cysteine is easily converted into glutathione in your body. It is possible to take glutathione itself in supplement form, although studies have shown it tends to get digested into its components and doesn't raise blood levels of glutathione as well as n-acetyl cysteine dose.

The sulfur in glutathione makes it sticky, and therefore glutathione acts a bit like sticky tape in your body; grabbing toxins and taking them out of your body. Glutathione also protects the antioxidant vitamins and minerals in your body; enabling them to last longer in your body, and continue protecting you from free radicals. As explained in chapter three, a number of different environmental chemicals and heavy metals have the ability to trigger an autoimmune disease in a genetically susceptible person. If you don't have optimal glutathione levels in your body, these nasty chemicals can persist longer in your body, stressing and over stimulating your immune system and raising inflammation.

Illness, ageing, nutrient deficiencies (particularly selenium and vitamin C), stress and toxicity can all deplete your body of glutathione. Once depleted, you are at higher risk of a flare up of an autoimmune disease, but also have a higher risk of cancer. Some research has shown that the lower your body's level of glutathione, the more severe your autoimmune disease is likely to be. One study showed low plasma glutathione to correlate strongly with severity of systemic lupus erythematosis[61].

Glutathione also helps to protect the liver from inflammation. This is beneficial for all autoimmune diseases, but particularly ones that target the liver specifically, and for people who have a fatty liver. Unfortunately, blood tests for glutathione are not readily available through pathology companies.

If you have an autoimmune disease, you are best off taking both Selenomune and n-acetyl cysteine in supplement form and watching for an improvement in symptoms or reduction in flare ups of your disease. That's the best way to judge how deficient in glutathione you may be. The average recommended dose of n-acetyl cysteine is 500mg to 1.5 grams daily. It should be taken on an empty stomach, away from food.

Zinc

Zinc is a mineral that is relied on by more than 200 enzyme systems in the body. Zinc is very important for a healthy immune system and for tissue repair. Having adequate levels of zinc in your body can help to prevent viral and bacterial infections and can help you overcome chronic viral infections such as glandular fever, mycoplasma and the other infections discussed in chapter three. Along with selenium, zinc can inhibit the replication of viruses. If your immune system is chronically stimulated by a long standing viral infection, you are more likely to develop an autoimmune disease and it's probably going to be more severe. Long standing viral infections are also very exhausting, therefore supplementing with zinc and other nutrients can help to give you back some energy.

Zinc plays an important role in tissue healing and repair, and that's why it's so important for anyone with a leaky gut; which is everyone with an autoimmune disease. Research has shown that zinc reduces the spaces between the tight junctions in the lining of the small intestine and hastens tissue repair after diarrhea or inflammation in the intestines[62]. Studies have shown that being zinc deficient increases the risk of suffering with intestinal parasites[63]. It is difficult to absorb zinc if you have a leaky gut and if you don't produce sufficient hydrochloric acid in your stomach.

Zinc is found in seafood (especially oysters), red meat, poultry and organ meat. The recommended dose of zinc in supplement form is between 30 and 60 milligrams per day.

Glutamine

Glutamine is well known for its ability to heal and seal a leaky gut. Glutamine is the most abundant amino acid in your bloodstream and is also found in high quantities in various tissues, including the gastrointestinal tract, liver, skeletal muscle, the brain and lungs. Your small intestine uses more glutamine than any other organ[64].

Glutamine assists in the proliferation and repair of intestinal cells and is the preferred fuel source for enterocytes (cells that make up the delicate lining of the small intestine).

Glutamine helps to strengthen tight junctions between intestinal cells and maintains the integrity of the intestinal lining

Glutamine helps to maintain GALT (Gut Associated Lymphoid Tissue, which is the immune system in your intestines), and secretory IgA.

Secretory IgA is the most abundant immunoglobulin in the lining of your small intestine and is vital for the function of the intestinal immune system. It provides an antiseptic paint to the lining of your small intestine and helps to prevent harmful bacteria from travelling across your gut lining, inflaming your gut and stimulating your immune system[65].

Glutamine helps to nourish the immune cells in your gut, which include fibroblasts, lymphocytes, and macrophages[66].

Lastly, glutamine is an essential component of the powerful antioxidant glutathione, necessary for detoxification and reducing inflammation.

An ideal dose of glutamine is between 2 and 4 grams per day.

MSM (Methyl Sulphonyl Methane)

MSM is a natural form of organic sulfur that is easily absorbed and used by the body. Sulfur is required for the maintenance of healthy connective tissue. MSM helps keep skin, hair and nails healthy by donating sulfur for the production of keratin. MSM also supports joint function and can help to reduce pain in all autoimmune diseases that affect the joints. It can also help to promote healing of joints that have been damaged by autoimmune disease, thereby reducing the risk of joint deformities and requirement for joint replacement.

Sulfur is also required for the function of the enzymes that carry out phase two detoxification in the liver. Phase two detox reactions are often inefficient because of poor liver health. This allows the accumulation of highly reactive and damaging toxins in the liver, which can cause damage to liver cells and elevated liver enzymes. Sulfur helps to improve the efficiency of liver detoxification, and it also reduces the risk of scar tissue from developing inside the liver. MSM works well when combined with vitamin C and a typical dose is 1 to 2 grams per day.

Bupleurum falcatum

Bupleurum is one of the most popular liver herbs used in traditional Chinese medicine. It has anti-inflammatory and hepatoprotective effects. That means it helps to protect liver cells from harm caused by inflammatory chemicals. This is very worthwhile because damaged liver cells spew out a host of inflammatory chemicals into the bloodstream. If we can reduce inflammation, it means we'll reduce symptoms of autoimmunity.

Studies have shown that bupleurum can potentiate the activity of cortisone[67].

That means if you are taking steroids like prednisone in the management of your disease, taking bupleurum may enable you to reduce your dose. That could help to minimise some of the harmful side effects of long term steroid use. Please don't alter your dose of medication unless you've discussed it with your doctor. Bupleurum has mild sedative properties and may help improve your quality of sleep if you struggle in this area. You can find bupleurum in supplement form in health food stores.

Berberine

Berberine is a natural plant extract, found in several different herbs. Examples include Goldenseal, Barberry and Phellodendron. It has a long tradition of use in Chinese Herbal Medicine. It has the following benefits:

- anti-inflammatory
- helps to heal a leaky gut
- anti-microbial
- anti-diabetic
- helps to lower cholesterol

Berberine is very useful for improving intestinal health in everyone with autoimmune disease. It has the ability to kill a range of different pathogens and is strongly recommended for anyone dealing with a parasitic gut infection or SIBO (Small Intestinal Bacterial Overgrowth). It has shown efficacy against various bacterial strains, including cholera, giardia, shigella, and salmonella, along with staphylococcus, streptococcus, and clostridium[68, 69].

It also has anti-protozoal effects against Giardia lamblia, Trichomonas vaginalis and Leishmania donovani[70, 71].

Berberine has remarkable abilities to heal a leaky gut. It helps to strengthen tight junctions between cells of the small intestine, thereby reducing intestinal permeability. Berberine also protects gut cells from the damaging effects of bacterial endotoxins (such as lipopolysaccharide), and reduces the amount of lipopolysaccharide absorbed into the bloodstream and entering the liver[72].

In this way, it helps to protect the liver from the toxic effects of a leaky gut. This reduces the liver's production of highly inflammatory chemicals (cytokines). The net effect is a reduction in inflammation, less tissue destruction and less fatigue.

The recommended dose of berberine is 1000 to 2000 milligrams per day, taken in divided doses with meals.

Magnesium

There's no one who doesn't benefit from a magnesium supplement. 300 different enzymes in your body require magnesium, and it's necessary for energy production. Therefore, magnesium is wonderful for reducing fatigue.

Magnesium is very important for your nervous system and your muscles. It has a calming, relaxing effect and can help you achieve a deeper, better quality sleep at night. Good, solid sleep is extremely beneficial for your immune system. You use up more magnesium when you are stressed because stress hormones cause loss of magnesium through the urine. Alcohol, sugar, exercise and heavy perspiration also deplete your body of magnesium.

Magnesium is predominantly found in green vegetables, nuts and seeds however, soils around the world are notoriously depleted in magnesium, it is therefore almost impossible to get enough of this mineral through your diet. The most common symptoms of magnesium deficiency are muscle cramps, spasms and twitches; headaches, restless legs syndrome, heart palpitations, anxiety, PMS and poor quality sleep.

The metabolism of vitamin D depends on magnesium. Therefore, raising your vitamin D level (through supplementation or increased sun exposure) can deplete your stores of magnesium. It's not uncommon for patients to begin supplementing with vitamin D, and then a couple of months later to experience leg cramps at night, restless legs or muscle twitches. Increasing your vitamin D level is necessary and beneficial, but you usually need to supplement with magnesium as well.

In order to benefit from its relaxing properties, it's best to take magnesium with your evening meal. The recommended dose is 400 to 600 milligrams (mg) per day.

Probiotics

Probiotics are good bacteria that live in your intestines. Taking a good quality probiotic is critical when healing autoimmune disease. Approximately 80 percent of your immune system is in your intestines, and the types of microbes you have living in your gut have the greatest influence over your immune health. Probiotics help to regulate your immune system; helping to keep it balanced and responding appropriately. You want your immune system to attack and destroy invading pathogens, but you also want to tolerate your own organs and tissues and not mount an attack on your own body, or attack harmless substances like pollen or dust mites.

You can take a probiotic in capsule form or you can get probiotics from consuming fermented foods. The benefit of taking a supplement is you know exactly which strain you're getting, and in what quantity. Unfortunately, the really good probiotics can be very expensive. Ideally, you would take probiotics both ways: as a supplement in capsule form and in fermented foods.

We have listed the benefits of probiotics on page 85. If you are searching for a probiotic supplement to take, we recommend you choose one that contains several different strains of organisms (between 6 and 12 strains), and high numbers in each capsule [between 20 and 60 billion CFU (stands for Colony Forming Units)].

There are certain species of probiotics that improve T-regulatory immune cell function. They include bacillus species, which are found in soil-based organisms. Therefore, certain soil-based organism probiotics can be very helpful for those with autoimmune disease, as impaired T-regulatory cell function is what allows the destruction of self organs and tissues.

Omega 3 essential fatty acids

The omega 3 fats EPA and DHA are highly beneficial for anyone suffering with autoimmune disease or pain because they lower inflammation by reducing the production of inflammatory cytokines.

A study published in the Journal of the American College of Nutrition titled Omega 3 fatty acids in inflammation and autoimmune diseases concluded that "Many of the placebo-controlled trials of fish oil in chronic inflammatory diseases reveal significant benefit, including decreased disease activity and a lowered use of anti-inflammatory drugs". [73]

Not many people get enough of these good fats in their diet

Modern diets are far too high in omega 6 polyunsaturated fats because they are so abundant in modern foods. Omega 6 fats are found in vegetable oils such as sunflower, canola, cottonseed, corn oil, safflower, soybean and peanut oil. They are also found in the fat of animals that have been fed grains; for example grain fed beef, poultry and eggs. An excess of omega 6 fats in the diet is strongly correlated with higher levels of inflammation, depression, cardiovascular disease and cancer.

EPA and DHA are two omega 3 fats found in oily fish as well as fish or krill oil supplements. The precursor to these fats (alpha linolenic acid) is found in plant foods such as flaxseeds, walnuts, pecans and chia seeds. Unfortunately, the human body doesn't do a good job of converting alpha linolenic acid into EPA and DHA, therefore we recommend you take a supplement.

Even if you eat oily fish every day, such as sardines or herrings, a supplement should help to reduce symptoms of pain and inflammation

An omega 3 supplement is particularly beneficial for anyone suffering with joint pain or skin inflammation (eg. psoriasis). The recommended daily dose is 1.5 to 2 grams of EPA and 1 gram of DHA. Omega 3 fats thin the blood, therefore if you're taking blood thinning medication, please discuss the dose of fish oil with your doctor before commencing.

Vitamin A

Vitamin A has many important functions in your body. Your eyes require a lot of vitamin A and it's best known for helping you to see in the dark. Vitamin A is also required for tissue healing. It's important to get enough vitamin A if you want to heal a leaky gut.

Vitamin A is only found in animal foods; egg yolks, liver and oily fish are the richest sources. Beta-carotene is a precursor of vitamin A and it's found in carrots and other brightly coloured vegetables and fruits, as well as green vegetables like broccoli and spinach. Many people think they'll get enough vitamin A as long as they eat plenty of vegetables. This is not always the case. In fact, vitamin A insufficiency is quite common.

Work out of Newcastle University in the UK suggests that between 40 and 50 percent of Caucasians produce insufficient levels of an enzyme necessary to convert beta-carotene into the active form of vitamin A (retinol)[74]. Vitamin A is also required for healthy T-regulatory cell function, which calms down an overactive immune system. Other white blood cells require vitamin A for optimal function, including neutrophils, macrophages and natural killer cells.

Vitamin A and vitamin D share a common receptor. If you take lots of vitamin D while having insufficient levels of vitamin A in your body, you may inadvertently create a problem in the digestive tract that aggravates an autoimmune condition.

Many people worry about vitamin A being toxic. It is true that pregnant women should not take high doses in supplement form. However, the average autoimmune patient is far more likely to be deficient, which harms the immune system.

Unless you are pregnant or trying to conceive, you can take between 15,000 IU and 50,000 IU per day.

Vitamin C

Vitamin C doesn't get the credit it deserves. It seems to have become the forgotten vitamin, or boring vitamin, thought to only protect you against the common cold. We'd like you to know that vitamin C has far more benefits than that.

Vitamin C is required for the formation of glutathione, which, you may recall, is your body's own powerful antioxidant and detoxifier. Raising glutathione helps to reduce inflammation in your body. Vitamin C is also necessary for the formation of collagen and connective tissue. Thus, it helps to reduce tissue damage and assist tissue repair, particularly in autoimmune diseases that affect the connective tissue, such as lupus and scleroderma. It also helps to reduce the free radical damage, wear and tear to the body that occurs in anyone with an autoimmune disease, and which speeds up ageing.

Vitamin C is found in fruits and vegetables, particularly citrus fruit, kiwifruit, broccoli and red bell pepper, however, it is destroyed by heat (cooking), and quickly breaks down once a fruit is pulled off a tree or a vegetables is pulled out of the ground. Therefore, the produce you buy at the supermarket is often quite depleted already.

The more stressed you are, and the poorer your state of health, the more vitamin C you require. It is safe to take very high doses of vitamin C; the only adverse effect is diarrhea. You can avoid this by taking vitamin C in divided doses; so that means taking a small amount several times each day, rather than a large amount at once. Of course, if you are prone to constipation, taking a high dose of vitamin C (or magnesium) can fix that for you.

Vitamin C works very well when combined with MSM (natural sulfur) and silica and you can find this in powder form called Collagen Food. The recommended dose is one to two teaspoons per day.

Low dose naltrexone

Low dose naltrexone is a treatment that's gaining popularity in the treatment of autoimmune disease. It works very well at relieving symptoms in some people and has no effect in others. It's not something we routinely recommend; we have included it here just so you are aware of it, should you choose to try it. Naltrexone was originally used to help opiate and heroin addicts, as well as alcoholics withdraw, and works by blocking the receptors for opiate hormones in our body. Therefore, if a heroin addict shoots up, they wouldn't feel anything because the opiate receptors would be completely blocked. It is also used in the emergency department of hospitals because it can save a heroin addict from an overdose if given in time.

The problem with using naltrexone in addicts is it blocks opiate receptors so well that people can't experience any pleasure at all. We naturally produce opiates and other feel-good chemicals like endorphins in our bodies, and naltrexone can block their effects, leading to feelings of despondency.

Back in the 1980s it was discovered that using a very tiny dose of naltrexone; between 3 and 4.5 milligrams (this is less than one tenth the dose used in addicts) had beneficial effects on the immune system. Low dose naltrexone works by reducing the ability of immune cells to make inflammatory chemicals. Therefore, it is sometimes used in autoimmune disease, cancer and fibromyalgia.

Low dose naltrexone needs to be taken at night, since this is the time that most opiate production occurs in the body

By blocking opiate receptors with a tiny dose of medication, the body responds by increasing production of opiates and endorphins. These feel-good chemicals have beneficial effects on T-regulatory cells (a type of white blood cell), which help to prevent the immune system from attacking your own body. Low dose naltrexone may also lower Erythrocyte Sedimentation Rate (ESR); therefore, the net effect is lowered inflammation in the body. Thus it can be a helpful way to reduce symptoms and help a patient feel better, but it does not address the cause of the autoimmune disease.

Low dose naltrexone requires a doctor's prescription and you'll need to get it from a compounding pharmacy. An average dose is 3 mg.

Chapter Eight

Troubleshooting:

What to do when the recommendations aren't working

If you have been following the eating plan and supplement suggestions in this book for at least three months but you are not experiencing significant health improvements, this chapter is for you. In it we will describe the most common conditions that can block or hinder recovery and what to do about them.

You may have a parasitic gut infection

The word parasite means an organism that lives on and feeds off of another organism. Intestinal parasites are very common. You don't need to have travelled to a third world country to have one. These infections are pretty easy to acquire, particularly if you don't have enough good gut bugs to protect you against infections.

Intestinal parasites can cause a great deal of inflammation to your gut lining. They can give you a very leaky gut, and the toxins these organisms produce can travel to your liver and make you feel really terrible.

Which parasites cause gut infections?

The following organisms are the most common culprits:

- Salmonella.
- Campylobacter.
- Shigella.
- Yersinia enterocolitica.
- Aeromonas.

- Giardia.
- Entamoeba histolytica.
- Dientamoeba.
- Blastocystis.
- Cryptosporidium.
- Clostridium difficile.
- Worms, including roundworms, tapeworms, pinworms, whipworms and hookworms.

What are the symptoms of a parasitic gut infection?

There are numerous. The following are the most common:

- Symptoms of irritable bowel syndrome such as bloating, diarrhea, constipation or gas.

- History of food poisoning or gastroenteritis and never feeling normal since.

- Feeling hungry soon after meals and like you are never really satisfied after eating.

- Poor quality sleep. Trouble getting to sleep, or frequent waking throughout the night; grinding your teeth at night or waking in the middle of the night with intense anxiety.

- Aching muscles or joints.

- Depression, anxiety, low motivation or foggy head.

- Fatigue.

- Iron deficiency.

- An itchy anus, particularly at night.

Well, after reading that list you probably want to rush out and get tested. That's a good idea because parasites are common, they are a common cause of continued poor health despite a good diet, and they can be treated.

Parasites are spread very easily and that's why it's important to wash your hands regularly, especially after using the bathroom, before eating and after touching animals

The best test for parasites is a stool test called "faecal MCS and PCR" test. MSC stands for Microscopy, Culture and Sensitivity, while PCR stands for Polymerase Chain Reaction (it tests for DNA fragments of microbes, therefore is highly sensitive). Your doctor can give you a referral for this test and it is covered by Medicare.

How to treat parasitic gut infections

These infections can be stubborn, and commonly used antibiotics are not always effective. There are some brilliant herbal remedies and essential oils but they are most effective when combined with the diet recommendations in this book and the recommendations for treating leaky gut in chapter four.

An unhealthy gut is a good home for parasites; therefore we must change the terrain; i.e. improve the health of your gut so it's no longer an appropriate home for parasites.

Conventional medicine uses a number of different antibiotics and anthelmintics (worming tablets) in the treatment of parasitic gut infections. The most commonly used drugs include Metronizadole (Flagyl), cotrimoxazole (Bactrim), nitazoxanide and paromomycin. These drugs are not always effective because the microbes are developing resistance to them.

Natural treatments for parasitic gut infections are usually far more effective. We recommend the following strategies:

- Follow the diet guidelines in chapter six of this book.

- Don't snack. Just eat three meals a day in order to give your digestive system a rest and to promote cleansing waves, which propel bacteria and other microbes downwards; enabling easier eradication.

- Take a Saccharomyces boulardii supplement. This is a beneficial yeast which promotes production of secretory IgA in the intestines. Secretory IgA has antiseptic properties. Saccharomyces boulardii also reduces inflammation in the gut by reducing production of the inflammatory chemical called interleukin 8.

- There are several very effective herbal antimicrobials, including berberine, oregano oil, thyme oil, clove oil and garlic.

- Take a good quality probiotic to strengthen the immune system and heal the tissue of the intestines.

- It is vital to heal the lining of the intestines with glutamine, bone broth, zinc and vitamin A.

Histamine intolerance

Histamine is a chemical produced in your body and related to immune system function. You have probably heard of histamine in relation to allergies and the use of antihistamine medication.

Histamine actually performs a range of important functions in your body, including healthy digestion and nervous system function. It is required for the production of stomach acid and it is a neurotransmitter (brain chemical).

If something like an allergy or insect sting irritates your immune system, histamine causes your blood vessels to dilate, enabling your white blood cells to quickly find and attack the problem.

> *A build up of histamine can give you a headache and leave you feeling flushed, itchy and tired*

This is a normal part of your body's natural immune response, but if you don't break down histamine properly, you can develop histamine intolerance.

The most common symptoms of histamine intolerance include:

- headaches or migraines
- anxiety
- problems falling asleep, or having very light sleep
- dizziness
- high blood pressure
- abnormally fast heart rate
- nausea
- abdominal cramps
- disrupted menstrual cycle
- facial flushing, especially after just one glass of fermented alcohol such as wine, champagne or beer
- blocked nose
- hives

The problem can result from too much histamine being produced inside your body; not being able to break down histamine properly, or from consuming more histamine-rich foods than your body can tolerate.

Foods very high in histamine include:

- Fermented alcohol, such as wine, beer and champagne
- Fermented foods such as sauerkraut, kimchi, kefir and kombucha, vinegar, soy sauce, yogurt
- Aged cheese
- Cured meats: bacon, hot dogs, salami, pepperoni, luncheon meats
- Citrus fruits
- Avocados
- Sourdough bread
- Smoked fish
- Eggplant, spinach, tomatoes
- Dried fruit

Some foods trigger your body to produce more histamine, and they include alcohol, bananas, nuts, strawberries, shellfish, chocolate and many artificial food colours and preservatives.

Alcohol and tea have the ability to block the enzyme that breaks down histamine, which is called diamine oxidase. If you have introduced fermented vegetables into your diet and you are feeling worse, histamine intolerance is the most likely culprit.

The most common cause of histamine intolerance is having low levels of the enzyme that breaks down histamine. Factors that reduce diamine oxidase production include:

- Gluten intolerance.

- SIBO (Small Intestinal Bacterial Overgrowth).

- Leaky gut.

- An inflamed digestive tract, caused by celiac disease or inflammatory bowel disease.

- Some people have inherited a genetic condition that impairs their ability to make the diamine oxidase enzyme. This is most common in Asian people.

- Several different medications can deplete this enzyme, including non-steroidal anti-inflammatory drugs (aspirin, ibuprofen), some antidepressants, some immune modifying drugs (Humira, Enbrel), antihistamines, some medication for abnormal heart rhythms and H2 histamine blockers (drugs used for blocking stomach acid, such as Zantac, Tagamet and Pepcid).

The best way to find out if you have histamine intolerance, is to avoid the foods high in histamine, as well as all alcohol and tea, and watch for an improvement in symptoms. You can also buy the enzyme responsible for breaking down histamine in supplement form. The enzyme is diamine oxidase. If taking this enzyme makes you feel significantly better, you are probably histamine intolerant.

The most important way to improve histamine tolerance though, is to fix your digestion; specifically improve the health of your small intestine. Following our recommendations for overcoming leaky gut in chapter four should help. Work on healing your gut, stay away from high histamine foods for around three months, and then you should find that your tolerance improves.

What to do if cravings get out of control

The diet we recommend for reversing autoimmune disease is quite restrictive and you may find it difficult to stick with. Please remember that it's not a forever diet. It is a means to an end. It is designed to reduce inflammation in your body as quickly as possible, to have you feeling better as fast as possible. To enable you to feel as good as you're supposed to feel and deserve to feel.

This is a low carbohydrate diet, and a sugar free diet. Many people find sugar quite addictive; if you've been eating it for a long time and then suddenly stop; your body will probably miss it. There are a number of reasons why you may be craving sugar. Understanding the mechanism may help you stick to the diet. Understanding the biological reasons for cravings is helpful because you'll know that it's not because you're a weak person who lacks willpower.

Common reasons for sugar and/or carbohydrate cravings include:

- Withdrawal symptoms. A lot of research has shown sugar to be quite addictive for many people. Eating it can light up your brain like a Christmas tree; encouraging the production of feel-good brain chemicals. Therefore, it's common to experience some temporary depression or anxiety after stopping sugar.

- Gut dysbiosis is a common cause of cravings. In nature it's a battle for survival. Certain harmful gut microbes have a high requirement for sugar. They depend on you eating sugar for their survival. There was an interesting article in The Atlantic titled "Your gut bacteria want you to eat a cupcake", which explained this well. Don't let the bad guys win! By avoiding sugar, you are depriving them of their fuel source and they will die. It helps to keep this in mind.

- Some people experience increased fatigue, cravings, headaches, aches and pains as symptoms of detoxification and as a die-off reaction when harmful yeast and microbes are dying in large numbers. These symptoms are temporary and you can help them to pass more quickly by drinking lots of water, green tea, supporting your liver health and taking activated charcoal capsules.

- Exhaustion, inadequate sleep and poor quality sleep are all common causes of cravings. Try to recognise these symptoms for what they are. What you really want is rest, not a biscuit.

- It takes a while for your body to adapt to using fat for energy instead of primarily glucose. Most people in society are sugar burners rather than fat burners. That means they derive most of their energy from carbohydrate. This is easy to achieve if you follow the standard diet, which is a high carbohydrate diet. If your body is accustomed to a regular intake of grains, cereals, starches and sugar, you will utilise them for energy. You will probably experience more hunger and won't be able to go long periods of time without food. This is because a high carbohydrate intake promotes high blood insulin levels, which suppress the fat burning hormones in your body. So you may have plenty (or surplus) body fat, yet you are starving and want to eat carbohydrate. It's a bit like a huge petrol tanker running out of fuel on the highway. It's full of fuel, but it just doesn't have access to it. Our eating plan in chapter six is lower in carbohydrate and higher in fat, therefore encourages your body to switch from predominantly burning glucose to predominantly burning fat. It takes most people several weeks to make the switch. The benefits of burning fat include losing some weight if you need to, but also sustained energy throughout the day (no energy slump at 3pm) and improved mental clarity.

- Deficiency of chromium and magnesium can promote sugar or carbohydrate cravings. You need these minerals in order to convert the food you've eaten into energy. You may find that supplementing with these nutrients significantly reduces carb cravings for you.

You may not believe us right now, but the good news is cravings will diminish the longer you follow our eating plan. Here are some suggestions for reducing their intensity:

- Make sure you are eating enough food at each meal. Since we discourage snacking, it's important for each meal to be filling and satisfying for several hours. Of course, you can snack if you're really feeling hungry and we've given you some healthy snack options on page 167. Please just don't snack as a habit.

- Make sure you are eating enough protein and healthy fats, as they are the most satiating nutrients. You may not be accustomed to eating fat, particularly if you've struggled with your weight for some time. Fat is very good for you, and the right fats, when consumed in the context of a lower carbohydrate diet, will actually make your metabolism more efficient and help you lose weight.

- You may need to consume more salt. Good quality salt is good for your , helping to improve adrenal gland exhaustion. People with adrenal gland exhaustion are more likely to experience sugar or salt cravings. If you're struggling with cravings for potato or corn chips, you definitely need to add more salt to your meals (and don't forget that chips are full of carbohydrate, not just salt). Please choose an unrefined salt, such as sea salt, Celtic salt or Himalayan salt. A lower carbohydrate diet has a mild diuretic effect, therefore a higher salt intake becomes necessary.

- Glutamine can help to reduce sugar cravings. You are probably already taking a glutamine supplement to help heal your gut, but if not, you may be interested to know that it helps carb cravings.

Glutamine can provide a quick source of fuel for your brain cells. Taking a teaspoon of glutamine can provide your brain with energy and can kill a carbohydrate craving within 15 minutes.

How to overcome adrenal gland exhaustion

Adrenal gland exhaustion is extremely common in people with autoimmune disease. In fact, almost everyone will have some degree of adrenal exhaustion. This makes sense because illness is a major stress on the body, and coupled with emotional stress, poor quality sleep and just the stress inherent in everyday life, it's no wonder the poor adrenal glands become overwhelmed.

Your adrenal glands manufacture the hormone cortisol. Cortisol levels fluctuate during the day in a circadian rhythm. It's supposed to be highest in the morning, in order to give you some energy, get you moving and inspired and it's supposed to drop in the evening, enabling you to unwind, get to sleep and stay asleep.

Many people with autoimmune disease have a disturbed cortisol rhythm; it tends to remain more or less at the same level all day, or it can rise in the evening, hindering good sleep.

This can leave you feeling tired and drained first thing in the morning when you get out of bed, yet unable to get to sleep or stay asleep in the evening

When the adrenal glands become exhausted, they can no longer pump out enough cortisol. Low cortisol tends to go hand in hand with low DHEA. These hormones can be measured in a blood test.

Cortisol should be checked twice; once at around 7:30 to 8am and again around 5 to 5:30pm.

Symptoms of adrenal gland exhaustion include:

- Dizziness, lightheadedness and/or fainting
- Low blood pressure
- Low blood sugar levels
- Brown pigmentation of the skin
- Depression, especially in the mornings
- Increased aches and pains
- Fatigue and exhaustion
- Waking up fatigued
- Light, broken sleep at night
- Feeling most energetic in the evening
- Cravings for sweet or salty foods
- Loss of libido
- Feeling rundown and catching infections frequently
- Tired and achy muscles
- Fibromyalgia
- Feeling stressed and easily overwhelmed
- Difficulty concentrating, foggy brain
- Sensitivity to cold

Many of the symptoms of adrenal exhaustion are the same as hypothyroidism (under active thyroid gland) and chronic fatigue syndrome. It is important to rule out other potential causes of these symptoms.

A number of things can help to restore adrenal gland health:

- Vitamin C, magnesium and B vitamins are all required by your adrenal glands. In fact, most of the vitamin C in your body is in your adrenal glands. The more stressed you are, the more of these nutrients your body requires. The best way to start feeling better as quickly as possible is to take these nutrients in supplement form.

- Get some exercise but don't push yourself too hard. Over exercising causes the adrenal glands to release cortisol. This would be a backward step in trying to overcome adrenal gland exhaustion. Listen to your body. Exercise to the point where it energises you, not exhausts you.

- Make sleep a priority. Try to get to bed by 10pm most evenings. If you feel like you need a nap during the day on weekends, take one. Sleep is extremely healing to your immune system, adrenal glands and every other part of your body.

- Meditation, yoga, journal writing and other relaxing activities help to reduce the effects of stress on your body.

- Your adrenal glands contain quite a lot of fat compared to other organs. Therefore, it's important to eat good amounts of healthy fats, to ensure their healthy function. Low fat diets are harmful to many organs of your body, including your adrenal glands.

- There are specific herbs that help to protect and restore the adrenal glands; they include tulsi, withania, rehmania, Siberian ginseng and Panax ginseng. They are available in supplement form.

If your blood DHEA levels are low or if chronic fatigue symptoms persist, taking DHEA can produce dramatically beneficial results. DHEA is a natural steroid hormone produced by healthy adrenal glands. It helps to improve energy, stamina and endurance.

How to handle an autoimmune flare

It's a fact of life that people with autoimmune disease typically have good days and bad days, or good weeks and bad weeks. It's natural to experience a flare up every so often; that's just the nature of the disease. Flare ups are commonly caused by stress, lack of sleep and infections. Sometimes you can't identify why the flare occurred.

While following the eating plan in this book, you may feel immensely better initially, but then experience a worsening of your symptoms for no good reason, even while you're sticking to the diet. Please keep going and don't get discouraged. What we are looking for in restoring your health is a general trend towards reduced symptoms and improved energy. Sometimes it takes several months to notice this pattern.

If you have been struck down with a flare up of your condition, the following strategies should help:

- **Sleep as much as possible.** Ideally you would go to bed and rest or try to have a nap. Sometimes the pain and inflammation prevent you from being able to sleep, but even closing your eyes and resting will help.

- **The quickest way to overcome an autoimmune flare is to fast (i.e. not eat).** However, this is not always practical or safe, especially if you have to keep working and driving. Fasting helps because it gives your digestive system a rest. Eating creates a great deal of oxidative stress and inflammation in anyone's body, let alone someone with leaky gut, SIBO and enzyme insufficiency, which is typical in autoimmune disease. Maybe you could have one day where you eat lightly and just drink vegetable juice, or smoothies and have bone broth; which brings us to our next point.

- **Drink bone broth.** Hopefully you include bone broth in your diet regularly; please see page 158 for its benefits. Bone broth is rich in minerals, gelatin, and other nutrients that are healing and soothing to your digestive system and nourishing for your entire body. It is quite safe for most people to do a modified fast where you only consume juices or smoothies, bone broth, fermented vegetables and coconut oil. If you just stick to those foods for a few days you'll probably find that the inflammation in your body subsides very quickly and the flare passes faster than it normally would.

- **Take serrapeptase.** Serrapeptase is an enzyme that was first discovered in the intestine of silkworms. This enzyme is necessary in order for the silkworm to dissolve the hard cocoon it is surrounded by, when it is ready to emerge as a moth. The silkworm also uses this enzyme to allow it to feed on tough mulberry leaves. These days, serrapeptase supplements are not derived from silkworms; the enzyme is derived from a natural fermentation process. Serrapeptase is a protease enzyme; that means it has the ability to digest protein. Research has shown this remarkable enzyme can help to dissolve non-living tissue in the body such as cysts, swellings, plaque and scar tissue. Serrapeptase is also wonderful for reducing inflammation in the body, thereby reducing pain and swelling, particularly in joints and muscles. Serrapeptase needs to be taken on an empty stomach.

- **Take an epsom salts bath.** Epsom salts contain magnesium, which is wonderful for helping to relax the body and relieve muscle aches and pains. Also, the sulphate found in epsom salts is very detoxifying. Epsom salt baths can improve the health of your lymphatic system and immune system. If you don't have the time for a full body bath, a foot bath can be almost as good. Put half a cup of epsom salts in a bucket of warm water while you sit and relax for half an hour. If you do this before bed you should have a much better sleep.

- **Take an activated charcoal supplement.** Activated charcoal may help by binding with the offending food, bacterial or fungal toxins in the intestines and preventing them from being absorbed by the body. Activated charcoal can bind with medications, so make sure you take it two hours away from medication or supplements. Make sure you drink plenty of water and take a magnesium supplement to prevent constipation.

Chapter Nine

Tests required in the diagnosis and monitoring of autoimmune disease

If you've been diagnosed with an autoimmune disease, chances are your doctor has ordered some or all of the following tests for you. Tests are necessary to define a disease and they are extremely useful for monitoring the disease. You can compare your test results before starting the protocol in this book with the results six months afterwards.

Most people find it extremely motivating and rewarding to be able to see the results of their efforts in black and white. Regular testing also means potential problems can be caught at an early stage, before serious harm can manifest.

Tests

Complete blood count

This test checks the quantity of red and white blood cells in your bloodstream, as well as the shape of your red blood cells. Abnormalities in red blood cells can indicate anaemia, which is common in people with autoimmune disease and people with malabsorption.

Low levels of a specific type of white blood cell called neutrophils is common in several types of autoimmune diseases and it is often an indicator of nutrient deficiencies.

Erythrocyte Sedimentation Rate (ESR)

This test measures the rate at which your red blood cells sediment (clump together). It is an indicator of how much inflammation is present in your body. It is a non-specific test, in that it tells us there is a lot of inflammation in the body, but not where the inflammation is coming from. It's a useful test to have done a few months after beginning the recommendations in this book because you should see your level plummet if it has been elevated.

The normal range for ESR is 1 - 28 mm/h.

High sensitivity C-reactive protein

C-reactive protein is made in your liver and it's an indicator of inflammation in your body. Again, it doesn't tell us where the inflammation is coming from. It can be raised due to autoimmune disease, infection, obesity, inflammatory disease or cancer. It is a useful way to monitor improvements in your condition because it improves more quickly than ESR.

The normal range for hs-C-reactive protein is 0.2 - 3 mg/L.

Liver function test

This is a very important test for monitoring the health of your liver. It measures the levels of specific enzymes that belong in your liver cells. If your liver cells become damaged for whatever reason, the enzymes leak into the bloodstream and give an elevated reading on a blood test. It also measures levels of bilirubin and proteins made by the liver.

People with autoimmune liver disease experience abnormalities in liver function, but liver inflammation is common in various different autoimmune diseases, particularly connective tissue diseases such as lupus.

> *Sometimes a bad case of leaky gut and dysbiosis can cause elevated liver enzymes, as the toxins spilling from the gut inflame the liver cells*

The normal reference ranges for a liver function test are as follows:

Total Bilirubin ....3 - 15 umol/L

Alk Phos...20 - 105 U/L

Gamma GT...5 - 35 U/L

LDH... 120 - 250 U/L

AST...0 - 35 U/L

ALT...5 - 30 U/L

Total Protein....................................64 - 83 g/L

Albumin...36 - 47 g/L

Globulin ....23 - 39 g/L

Kidney function test

Monitoring kidney function is very important for anyone with connective tissue disease, such as lupus. It is also important for monitoring potential drug side effects.

A kidney function test checks for levels of electrolytes, waste products of protein break down, and the rate at which your kidneys filter your blood (Glomerular filtration rate [eGFR]).

The following comprises a kidney function test:

Sodium.. 135 - 145 mmol/L

Potassium...3.5 - 5.5 mmol/L

Chloride ....95 - 110 mmol/L

Bicarbonate... 20 - 32 mmol/L

Urea ....3.0 - 8.0 mmol/L

Creatinine ....45 - 85 umol/L

eGFR... >59 mL/min/1.73m2

Thyroid Function Test

This test is most useful for those with Hashimoto's thyroiditis or Graves' disease, however there is a strong association with thyroid problems, celiac disease and lupus. If you are experiencing sustained fatigue, depression, fluid retention and an inability to lose weight, we strongly recommend you have your thyroid function checked. After all, autoimmune thyroid disease is the most common autoimmune disease in the world. The presence of thyroid antibodies is an early warning sign that autoimmune destruction is occurring to the thyroid gland, and if not halted, thyroid hormone abnormalities will follow. There is more information about thyroid conditions in our book, Your Thyroid Problems Solved.

We recommend the following thyroid tests:

TSH...0.3 - 2.5 mIU/L

free T4 ....8 - 22pmol/L

free T3...2.5 - 6.0 pmol/L

Thyroid antibodies

Thyroglobulin Ab.......................................0 - 40 IU/mL

 Thyroid Peroxidase Ab........................... 0 - 35 IU/mL

TSH receptor antibodies ....less than 1 IU/L

Cortisol

Cortisol is made by your adrenal glands and is produced in response to stress. High levels of cortisol can indicate extreme or long term stress and excess cortisol is often seen in those with insulin resistance (syndrome X), polycystic ovarian syndrome and women who carry excess weight in their abdominal area. Low cortisol is a feature of adrenal gland exhaustion.

Cortisol should be tested in the morning; approximately 7:30 am to 8:30 am and again in the afternoon, at approximately 5pm.

Morning cortisol should be between 200 and 650 nmol/L. Afternoon cortisol should be between 100 and 400 nmol/L.

DHEA-S

Dehydroepiandrosterone sulphate is made in your adrenal glands. The hormone has immune system benefits and improves energy levels and stamina. Low levels are commonly seen in people with long term illness or chronic fatigue syndrome. Elevated levels are typically seen in women with polycystic ovarian syndrome.

The normal range for women is 1 - 11 µmol/L

The normal range for men is 2.5 – 13.0 µmol/L

Vitamin D

This is probably the most important blood test for anyone affected by an autoimmune disease. Raising vitamin D is an extremely easy and effective way of reducing the level of inflammation in your body. It also greatly reduces your risk of coming down with an infection. Chronic, lingering infections that pathologically stimulate the immune system can often be resolved by improving vitamin D status, along with other nutrients and diet changes.

There are two different vitamin D tests. The most common vitamin D blood test is called 25 hydroxy vitamin D, or 25 (OH) Vitamin D3. The ideal level in the bloodstream for optimal immune system health is between 40 and 80 ng/mL. However, this is the inactive form of vitamin D in your blood. The biologically active form is called 1,25 (OH) vitamin D.

Sometimes it's necessary to have both forms tested. Our kidneys convert inactive vitamin D to its active form. Magnesium is required for that conversion. Magnesium insufficiency is very common.

Various medications, including steroids, diuretics and stomach acid blocking drugs can deplete the body of magnesium. Impaired kidney function can also hinder activation of vitamin D. Sometimes, supplementing with vitamin D can result in a build up of the inactive form, and a deficiency of the active form. This can cause higher blood calcium levels and symptoms including nausea, heart palpitations, constipation, body aches, hyperparathyroidism and an increased risk of kidney stones.

When having a vitamin D blood test, it is best to have the following two tests:

1,25 (OH) Vitamin D3: Active Reference range is 13 - 46 pg/mL

25 (OH) Vitamin D3: Inactive Reference range is 40 - 80 ng/mL

It's important to remember that just because you take a vitamin D supplement, it doesn't mean you have sufficient levels of active vitamin D in your bloodstream.

If you have been taking a vitamin D supplement for some time but your blood tests are showing your level is still low, there is always an explanation. It is usually due to poor digestion, dysbiosis or chronic infection. If your blood test result shows low inactive vitamin D and high active vitamin D, it is often a sign of chronic infection. Resolving the infection usually resolves the vitamin D ratio[75].

Serum retinol

This is a blood test for vitamin A. Low levels of vitamin A are common in people with poor digestion, and particularly fat malabsorption, since vitamin A is fat soluble. Deficiency can also occur in people with the common genetic condition where beta carotene is not converted into vitamin A efficiently enough in the body. This is especially common in Caucasians, affecting approximately 40 percent[76].

The normal range is 0.7-2.8 µmol/L.

Serum folate

This measures the amount of folate (folic acid) in your blood. The normal level is greater than 7.0 nmol/L.

Serum vitamin B12

The normal amount of vitamin B12 to have in your bloodstream is 180 - 740 pmol/L. Low levels of vitamin B12 are very common in people with digestive problems. It is quite difficult to absorb B12 from foods, therefore, it's one of the first nutrient deficiencies that occurs when there is poor digestion. Low stomach acid and small intestinal bacterial overgrowth are often present in people with low B12 or low-normal. The autoimmune disease pernicious anaemia produces significant vitamin B12 deficiency.

An ideal level is at least 400 pmol/L.

Homocysteine blood test

This test is a useful indicator of how well you utilise folate and vitamin B12 in your body. If you are deficient in these B vitamins, or not activating and utilising them correctly, your blood homocysteine level will rise. Elevated homocysteine is related to an increased risk of numerous health problems, including heart attacks, strokes, infertility and depression.

The normal level of homocysteine is 5 - 15 umol/L.

Iron

A blood test called iron studies is the most thorough test of your body's iron status. It encompasses a ferritin test, which indicates how much iron is stored in your body, particularly your liver. A normal ferritin level is considered to be between 20 and 200 ug/L. Ideally it should be above 50. Low iron is very common in people with small intestinal bacterial overgrowth and other digestive problems.

Secretory IgA

Secretory IgA (sIgA) is a beneficial immune molecule secreted by the mucosal tissue lining the gastrointestinal tract. It helps to provide a protective barrier, keeping harmful microbes from being able to cause infection in the gut. People with low levels of secretory IgA are more prone to dysbiosis and parasitic gut infections. They are also more prone to cancer. Long standing inflammation to the lining of the gut, such as caused by celiac disease or a gut infection can cause a temporary elevation in secretory IgA.

Reference range = 0.69 - 3.09 g/L

ANA (Anti-Nuclear Antibodies)

This is a non-specific test to check for the presence of autoimmune disease. More than 95 percent of patients with lupus test positive for anti-nuclear antibodies, but they are found in many different autoimmune diseases, particularly those affecting the joints and connective tissue. A positive anti-nuclear antibody test warrants further blood tests to check for the presence of other auto-antibodies.

Anti ds (double stranded) DNA antibodies

This is a more specific blood test for systemic lupus erythematosus. In normal healthy people the level should be less than 5 IU/mL. There are a number of additional antibody tests used in the diagnosis of lupus and related connective tissue diseases.

Rheumatoid factor antibody

This antibody is found in the blood of approximately 80 percent of people with rheumatoid arthritis. Higher levels correlate with greater disease severity. It is also present in the blood of people with other autoimmune diseases that affect the joints.

Chapter Ten

Case studies of patients who have reversed their autoimmune disease

Overcoming Graves' disease

Jacinta was 25 years old when she first came to see me for help with an over active thyroid gland. She had been diagnosed with Graves' disease two and a half year ago and had been taking the drug Neomercazole (carbimazole) for all that time. Neomercazole blocks the ability of the thyroid gland to manufacture hormones and, therefore, it's usually very effective for controlling Graves' disease.

Jacinta was only taking a small dose of Neomercazole (one tablet twice daily). However, her doctor stressed the fact that it's not ideal to take this medication long term and he was trying to convince her to have her thyroid gland removed. Jacinta wanted to avoid that at all costs, and that's why she came to our clinic.

I asked Jacinta to complete a thorough health questionnaire, and from that I learned she suffers with fatigue, hay fever and constipation. I asked Jacinta about her health history and she mentioned a particularly bad case of glandular fever that lingered for approximately three months. You may remember from chapter three that glandular fever is a common trigger of autoimmune disease. Jacinta's mum had had Graves' disease and her sister had type 1 diabetes, so Jacinta definitely had the genetic predisposition to develop an autoimmune disease.

Jacinta's thyroid hormones were all normal because she was taking Neomercazole. However, her TSH receptor antibodies were raised (6

IU/L). In Graves' disease, the immune cells produce antibodies that bind to TSH receptors on the thyroid gland and they trick the thyroid into producing sky high levels of hormones. Neomercazole is very useful for getting hormone levels under control, but it does nothing to address the underlying immune dysfunction that created the condition.

My recommendations for Jacinta

- Jacinta was following a gluten and dairy free diet most of the time, because of what she had read about leaky gut syndrome. I stressed the importance of sticking with this diet all of the time, as it usually takes several months for the inflammation caused by those foods to subside. I also asked Jacinta to remove soy milk and corn chips from her diet, as they can cause inflammation to the intestines.

- I checked Jacinta's blood vitamin D level and it was inadequate (25 ng/mL). I asked her to take 3000 IU of vitamin D each day with breakfast and asked her to spend some time in the midday sun regularly but briefly.

- I asked Jacinta to take 200 mcg of Selenomune each day. Selenomune helps to reduce autoantibody production, therefore, is helpful for everyone with autoimmune disease.

- I gave Jacinta some fish oil capsules because they reduce inflammation and help to heal damaged tissue.

- I put Jacinta on the program in chapter six for healing leaky gut and helping her liver.

I didn't see Jacinta again for another year and a half. She told me she felt fantastic and was able to come off the Neomercazole with her doctor's supervision. Her TSH receptor antibodies had gone down to normal and the Graves' disease was in remission. Jacinta stayed off gluten; she ate a bit of cheese and yogurt occasionally; she ate corn chips occasionally and swapped the soy milk for almond milk. She was able to remain feeling very well on that eating plan for nearly a year.

Jacinta came back to see me because the Graves' disease was slowly returning. Her TSH level was starting to decline again and the TSH receptor antibodies were rising. She had lost almost 4 and a half pounds without trying and this is a common symptom of hyperthyroidism. Jacinta wanted to avoid going back on the Neomercazole.

I asked her several questions and found out she had stopped taking all of her supplements

It was winter at the time and when I checked her vitamin D level, it was only 19 ng/mL. Vitamin D is so important for keeping autoimmune disease at bay; an ideal level is between 40 and 80 ng/mL. Jacinta had been stressed; she had recently started a new job, and the job involved some shift work. For the first time in her life she was working nights for part of the week. She found it difficult to get to sleep and felt chronically sleep deprived. I asked Jacinta to take a magnesium supplement, which would calm her nervous system and help her get to sleep.

I repeated the same regime with Jacinta and emphasized the importance of taking the supplements, particularly vitamin D and Selenomune long term. I also added a small amount of iodine to her regime (160 mcg). She was able to prevent the onset of Graves' disease and has been feeling well for the previous two years.

Pre-autoimmune disease

Kimberly is a 52 year old lady who came to see me recently with a long list of health complaints. She had been feeling very unwell for the previous two years but no doctor actually diagnosed a particular disease. Kimberley suffered with extreme exhaustion. She underlined the word exhausted on her questionnaire. She said to me "There's a lot of stuff I didn't even write on the questionnaire. You're going to think I'm crazy when I tell you all my symptoms".

Kimberley was a teacher and had to cut down her work days from full time to two days a week. Headaches and neck pain were significant problems for Kimberley. She had a sore head and sore neck just about all the time. She tried not to take pain relievers but felt like she couldn't function without them on the two days she worked.

Kimberley suffered with one sinus infection after another and took several courses of antibiotics each year. Her nose was constantly blocked, her ears would pop and crackle and she continually had mucus dripping down the back of her throat.

Kimberley suffered with really awful digestive problems. She was constantly bloated and described herself as a gas factory. She had loose bowel motions that smelt so bad that she said her family all wanted to leave the house every time she used the bathroom. Kimberley also felt nauseous all the time, and the best way she found to relieve the nausea was to eat. So she snacked all day.

Kimberley was already taking several supplements: turmeric, St John's wort and magnesium. The turmeric and magnesium fixed the aches and pains she used to experience in just about every muscle of her body. The St John's wort greatly reduced the depression and anxiety she was prone to. If she tried to come off St John's wort she noticed an immediate severe decline in her mood.

As with many patients with autoimmune conditions, Kimberley had terrible sleep and she woke up feeling like a wreck

She woke around five times each night and it was sometimes hard to get back to sleep. Looking at her adrenal gland hormones, she had a mild case of adrenal gland exhaustion. Not surprising at all, considering everything her poor body was going through.

My recommendations for Kimberley

- Kimberley was a reader of our newsletters, so she tried to implement a lot of our recommendations. She was already avoiding gluten strictly and her diet wasn't too bad overall. Unfortunately, the constant eating due to nausea meant that her digestive system never had a rest between meals. It was having to deal with the hard work of digesting food all day long. All that food was fermenting inside her gut and creating a really toxic environment. Kimberley had the symptoms of SIBO (Small Intestinal Bacterial Overgrowth) and I put her on the stage 2 eating plan on page 167 to remedy that, along with the strategies to heal leaky gut on page 82.

- She needed a lot of digestive support, therefore I asked Kimberley to take digestive enzymes with each meal. She felt far less bloated and gassy when she took them.

- Blood tests confirmed that Kimberley was low in iron and vitamin D, as well as vitamin B12. This is really common for people with malabsorption and an overgrowth of harmful gut bugs. I gave Kimberley supplements and they lifted her energy levels very quickly.

- Magnesium helped Kimberley fall asleep and it also stopped the headaches. People with gut problems often have poor quality sleep because the endotoxins leak through the gut wall throughout the night and overwork the liver. The longer she stayed on our recommended plan, the better her sleep became.

I have seen Kimberley twice since her initial visit and her improvements have been remarkable. She said to me "I feel like I'm getting my life back. For so long I was just surviving; not living". I'm convinced that Kimberley would have gone on to develop one or more autoimmune diseases had she not decided to turn her life around.

Overcoming Rheumatoid Arthritis

Melita is a delightful 54 year old lady who came to see me for help with rheumatoid arthritis. She had been suffering with rheumatoid arthritis for 28 years and she had been taking the steroid prednisone for 28 years. The dose was fairly small (10 mg) most of the time. Her doctor raised the dose when she had a flare, which was approximately once a year.

The prednisone had contributed to insulin resistance (syndrome X/ pre-diabetes). This meant Melita struggled with her weight a lot and found it impossible to shift the excess weight around her torso. Her dad is a type 2 diabetic, which makes it likely Melita could go down the same path.

Apart from joint pain, Melita suffered with the following symptoms:

- Brain fog. Melita worked full time and found it increasingly difficult to focus and concentrate. She said "My mind is like a sieve. It's becoming really scary with the important things I'm forgetting".

- Depression, anxiety and a sense of panic. Melita was increasingly feeling overwhelmed and like she couldn't cope.

- Hot and cold sweats. These mostly occurred after eating. Melita had gone through an early menopause 10 years ago and she didn't feel like the sweats were related to that.

- Melita had been off gluten and dairy products for 10 years but she still suffered with nausea and reflux.

- Melita had an episode of post-partum thyroiditis after the birth of her second child 21 years ago. She was on a very low dose of thyroxine for a year and then the condition resolved itself. Post-partum thyroiditis is autoimmune.

Melita had a strong family history of autoimmune disease; her brother has vitiligo and type 1 diabetes. Her mum has ITP (Idiopathic Thrombocytopenia) and a cousin has Hashimoto's thyroiditis.

I was very excited when Melita came to see me because I knew we could do something to help her feel a lot better

Melita's diet was very good, although I asked her to make some adjustments:

- She ate a lot of vegetables, which was wonderful, but she didn't eat much protein or healthy fat. Because she was always trying to lose weight, she kept her portion sizes very small and there was barely any fat in her meals. This left her feeling hungry for much of the day and consequently she snacked on dried fruit and nuts throughout the day. That wasn't conducive to weight loss or improved digestive health. Therefore, I asked her to increase her protein and fat portions and try not to snack during the day.

- Because of the nausea and reflux, I treated Melita for SIBO (Small Intestinal Bacterial Overgrowth) by putting her on the low FODMAP stage 2 eating plan on page 167. I also implemented the strategies to heal leaky gut and support her liver.

- Melita was already taking vitamin D and her blood level was good (46 ng/mL). She was taking magnesium but nowhere near enough. I switched her over to Magnesium Ultra Potent Powder and asked her to take a teaspoon with dinner each evening.

It was wonderful to see Melita eight weeks later because she felt so much better. The first thing she mentioned was how much better she felt emotionally. Because she felt so anxious all the time, Melita rarely went anywhere she didn't have to go. She didn't want to socialise and she felt apprehensive about going to places she hadn't been before. She actually said to me "I don't feel like that at all now. Now I feel confident and adventurous". I was so pleased to hear how much her quality of life had improved.

Melita had lost 13 pounds and she was thrilled with that because she could never get her weight to budge in the past. She no longer suffered with the hot and cold sweats and she was able to link that symptom to sugar. She said "I ate sugar three times since I last saw you and they were the only times I got the hot and cold sweats". Melita said her brain felt clear and it was so much easier to get her work done in the office. Her doctor had reduced her dose of prednisone with the plan of coming off it altogether.

Melita still wants to lose another 12 or 13 pounds and I've placed her on a ketogenic diet to help shift the remaining weight.

Healing Autoimmune Hepatitis

Greg was 48 when he came to our clinic seeking help for autoimmune hepatitis. He had been diagnosed six months ago and was desperately seeking answers. Greg first visited his doctor because he felt incredibly tired and no matter how much he slept, he still felt exhausted first thing in the morning, and for the rest of the day.

Greg's doctor ordered a blood test called a liver function test and Greg's liver enzymes were significantly raised. His results were as follows:

Total bilirubin 38

Alk. P 94

GGT 261

ALT 846

AST 507

LD 276

Greg went on to have a liver biopsy and the results showed "bridging necrosis" and "marked inflammation". There was "a severe interface and lobular hepatitis, which is autoimmune-like in pattern". The summary read "Severe portal and lobular hepatitis with early fibrosis".

Greg's liver was highly inflamed and was beginning to show early signs of scar tissue (cirrhosis). There was a period of time where Greg was seeing his specialist nearly every week for additional tests and monitoring of his condition. Greg was a highly motivated person. He owned a bicycle store and he did a lot of cycling in his spare time. He was willing to do whatever it took to make him well. The fatigue meant he had to cut down his hours at work and he was no longer able to go cycling.

Greg's diet wasn't fantastic. Because he was such a busy person, he often ate foods that are quick and convenient. He ate a lot of bread, breakfast cereal and muesli bars, and his favourite dinner was pasta. Because he was slim and fit, Greg thought he could get away with eating whatever he liked because he could just burn the calories off.

My recommendations for Greg

- Greg's vitamin D level was too low (23 ng/mL). He only got the chance to go out into the sun on weekends and that wasn't providing him with enough vitamin D. Also the liver is involved in vitamin D production and because his liver was so inflamed, it probably couldn't do the job well enough.

- I asked Greg to follow the stage one eating plan on page 164 and follow our guidelines for healing leaky gut and supporting the health of his liver. He took four capsules of LivaTone Plus each day, along with 200 mcg of Selenomune and two teaspoons of MSM powder each day.

- Greg took a high dose probiotic each day and four grams of glutamine powder every day. Although he never experienced any digestive problems, healing autoimmune disease involves healing the gut and improving the health of the immune system that resides within the intestines.

It took nearly two years but Greg was able to arrest the autoimmune disease and stop any further destruction to his liver. His liver enzymes all returned to normal and he regained his energy and ability to do 80 kilometre bike rides on weekends.

Reversing Multiple Sclerosis

Maria is a 60 year old lady who first came to our clinic around 18 months ago for help with multiple sclerosis. She was diagnosed with MS three months ago and her doctor put her straight on Interferon injections (Rebif). This drug is thought to slow the progression of MS but that's controversial and up for debate.

Maria first went to her doctor because of a strange sensation she had in her left leg, which eventually got so bad that she developed difficulties walking.

> *Subsequently she had an MRI scan of her brain which showed four distinct lesions consistent with a demyelinating process*

Maria was a believer in nutritional supplements and she came to see me for advice on which nutrients are most appropriate for her.

Maria was taking several nutritional supplements including magnesium and vitamin D. She couldn't be without the magnesium because it prevented her from getting leg cramps at night and improved the quality of her sleep. Maria wasn't taking enough vitamin D; she was only taking one capsule each day (1000 IU). This wasn't raising her blood level of vitamin D to where it should be. I asked her to take 5000 IU each day with breakfast or lunch and I planned to re test her blood in three months time.

My recommendations for Maria

- Maria is Italian and she loves bread. She would eat it at every meal if she could, but stops herself because it gives her mild indigestion and tends to make her gain a few pounds around the waist. It took some convincing to get Maria to follow a gluten and dairy free diet but she eventually agreed to give it a go.

- I put Maria on the leaky gut healing protocol in chapter four and gave her LivaTone Plus with turmeric to help support her liver. I also gave her n-acetyl cysteine for a more powerful anti-inflammatory effect.

- I gave Maria 200 mcg of Selenomune and asked her to take six high strength fish oil capsules each day, to reduce inflammation and help her immune system.

- I asked Maria to include a lot of good fats in her diet. The myelin sheath that gets attacked in MS is made of fat; therefore it's important to consume plenty of good fats to rebuild it. Examples of healthy fats include olive oil, avocados, coconut oil, nuts (especially macadamia nuts), seeds, ghee and the fat from pastured lamb and beef. She began eating more fat than she ever had in the past and, in the first month, lost six and a half pounds. In the context of a low carbohydrate diet, eating more fat can help you lose weight.

I saw Maria every month for quite some time. She was thrilled with how much better she felt and couldn't believe how much energy she had. Her sleep quality greatly improved and she now woke each morning feeling refreshed. Maria sticks to the diet most of the time; she likes to come in for regular visits for reinforcement.

She went on a one month holiday to stay with family in Italy and some gluten slipped back into her diet - she then experienced such bad indigestion which lasted nearly two weeks. At the same time, she noticed weakness in her left leg, which had not bothered her for a long time.

Maria saw her specialist every six months for a checkup. She had been able to reduce her dose of Interferon significantly and her doctor was extremely pleased with her progress. Maria had another MRI scan of her brain 10 months after her initial one at diagnosis.

This one was startlingly different. The first scan identified four lesions; this one only identified one

The report said the following:

"The previous examination showed a lesion within the cervical cord at the level of C2/3. This is visible on today's examination but is less conspicuous and barely seen on the sagittal series. The lesion has significantly reduced in size. No further definite cord lesion is seen".

Maria comes for a visit every three months or so because she says it helps to keep her focused on her health.

Healing Ulcerative Colitis

Leena is a 47 year old lady who came to see me for help with ulcerative colitis. She was in the middle of a flare and was really fed up with feeling so dreadful for so long. She had had ulcerative colitis for the previous five years and she experienced a flare up roughly every six months. She had been taking mesalazine (Mezavant) for five years and her doctor put her on prednisone every time she had a flare. Mesalazine is an anti-inflammatory drug which is a derivative of salicylic acid (the active ingredient in aspirin).

Things were pretty bad for Leena when she was having a flare up of ulcerative colitis; she had mucousy diarrhea approximately 15 times a day and she woke around 3am each morning, as that's when the diarrhea began for the day. She had broken sleep with abdominal cramps until 6am when she had to get ready for work. Not surprisingly, she was deeply exhausted all the time.

Leena dragged herself from one task to the next throughout the day

Leena was also overweight. She wanted to lose around 20 to 30 pounds. She felt quite helpless at achieving this because she definitely didn't have the energy to exercise, and in order to get through the day she snacked on chocolate. There was a lot of stress in Leena's life as she ran her own business.

Leena developed ITP (Idiopathic Thrombocytopenia, which is an autoimmune disease) when she was 22 years old. It was a mild case that cleared on its own, however her platelets remained on the very bottom of the normal range. Her mum has an under active thyroid gland caused by Hashimoto's thyroiditis and that's the only family history of autoimmune disease Leena is aware of.

Because Leena was such a busy person, she ate foods that are quick to swallow. Salads take too long to chew, so she lived on bread, crackers, cheese and yogurt. She did eat a good meal in the evening because she cooked for her husband and children. Leena drank a lot of wine. When filling out the questionnaire, in response to "How much alcohol do you drink?" she wrote "Too much". It's a problem because alcohol causes a leaky gut and promotes the growth or harmful gut microbes; two things that stand in the way of overcoming autoimmune disease.

My recommendations for Leena

- I explained the importance of healing leaky gut and supporting liver health to Leena. I placed her on the stage 2 eating plan in chapter six. Because her digestion was so poor, I removed high FODMAP foods from her diet because she had temporarily lost the ability to digest them. They were fermenting inside her and feeding all the wrong bacteria and yeast, which were inflaming her gut lining.

- Leena was low in vitamin D because she rarely went outside into the sunshine and because chronic diarrhea and leaky gut inhibits the absorption of fat soluble nutrients. I gave Leena supplements of vitamin D (5000 IU) and vitamin A (25,000 IU), to support her immune system, reduce inflammation and heal her gut lining.

- Leena needed a high dose of glutamine. It is wonderful for helping to heal a leaky gut, but also offers symptomatic relief for anyone suffering with chronic diarrhea or abdominal pain.

- I gave Leena a selenium supplement of 200mcg daily, as it helps to increase glutathione production and calm the immune system.

Leena responded to the diet changes very quickly. I saw her six weeks later and she was vastly improved. She had lost over 17 pounds, had much more energy and the diarrhea had stopped. It enabled her to come off the prednisone.

I saw Leena again in another four weeks and she had improved further. She said "I feel so good now, I can get on with my life".

She had been able to reintroduce high FODMAP vegetables and fruits back into her diet and tolerated them well. Unfortunately, she ate some peanut butter one night and spent most of the next day on the toilet. Leena was very sensitive to peanuts and also other legumes. She is managing her condition well and has been gradually reducing her dose of mesalazine.

Chapter Eleven

The Conventional medical treatment of autoimmune disease

It's quite likely that the reason you are reading this book is because you're unhappy with the treatment your doctor or specialist has offered you for your autoimmune disease.

Conventional medicine aims to block, suppress or inhibit the immune system and, in that way, reduce inflammation and tissue damage. The most commonly used drugs include steroids and TNF-Alpha Blockers (Tumour Necrosis Factor-Alpha Blockers). The TNF-Alpha Blockers are referred to as disease modifying drugs. They do suppress the immune system well but, unfortunately, also increase the risk of cancer and serious infections.

Chemotherapy drugs are sometimes used for autoimmune disease; the most common examples include methotrexate, Imuran and cyclosporine. In severe cases of disease, a bone marrow transplant is sometimes given.

Most of the drugs used for autoimmune disease have intense and serious side effects, particularly if used long term

One of the most common reasons patients come to our clinic is they can no longer stand the side effects of their medication; which isn't even controlling their disease particularly well.

If you are taking medication for autoimmune disease, this chapter may help you to understand how it works and will give you some information about side effects you may have experienced.

The following medications are commonly used for autoimmune disease:

Corticosteroids

Synthetic corticosteroids mimic the effects of natural corticosteroids produced in your own body and they are very powerful at reducing inflammation. They are often the first drug given in order to reduce inflammation quickly and stabilise the disease. The most commonly used corticosteroid is prednisone. Other corticosteroids include hydrocortisone, dexamethasone, and methylprednisolone.

Steroids have a lot of side effects, including:

- Easy bruising.
- Weight gain. They can cause a significant amount of weight gain in a very short space of time. They promote weight gain around the trunk in particular.
- Steroids strongly promote syndrome X (also known as insulin resistance, metabolic syndrome and pre-diabetes). In a person who is pre-diabetic, steroids can push them into full blown type 2 diabetes.
- Steroids can cause diabetics to experience a worsening of their disease; higher blood sugar and more complications.
- Increased hunger and cravings for carbohydrate and sugar.
- Psychological changes such as irritability or depression, and sometimes euphoria.
- Increased risk of cataracts.
- Fluid retention.
- Insomnia.
- Atrophy of the adrenal glands.
- Increased cholesterol and triglycerides.
- If used long term, steroids lead to bone loss and significantly raise the risk of osteoporosis.

Because of the numerous side effects, steroids are usually reserved for short term use. They are very effective at reducing inflammation, but once the disease is under control, the patient is slowly weaned off them.

Non-Steroidal Anti-Inflammatory Drugs (NSAIDs)

NSAIDs suppress inflammation and also have an analgesic (pain relieving) effect. They work by inhibiting the release of leukotrienes and prostaglandins, which are natural substances produced by your body that cause pain and inflammation. NSAIDs have quite a weak effect compared to the other drugs used for autoimmune disease. Examples of these drugs include aspirin, ibuprofen and naproxen.

Unfortunately these drugs cause a leaky gut, which is exactly what we don't want when treating autoimmune disease. If you need to use them occasionally, please take a teaspoon of glutamine at the same time to mitigate some of the intestinal damage. Also make sure you never take them on an empty stomach. Make sure you eat a good amount of protein at the same time.

Possible side effects include stomach upset, nausea, fluid retention; an increased risk of kidney damage, and increases in blood pressure and heart attack risk. High doses are capable of causing gastrointestinal bleeding.

Some autoimmune diseases make the blood thick and sticky and prone to clots.

In those instances a small dose of aspirin taken long term can greatly reduce the risk of blood clots and it is very helpful in managing the disease.

Anti-malarial drugs

More than 50 years ago it was discovered that anti-malarial drugs have a mild immuno-suppressive effect, therefore are useful for some autoimmune diseases. These drugs are most commonly used for lupus and rheumatoid arthritis and they can reduce inflammation in the lining of the lung (pleurisy) and heart (pericarditis), as well as improve joint and muscle pain. These drugs also reduce fever and fatigue. The most commonly used antimalarial drug is hydroxychloroquine (Plaquenil).

Possible side effects include:

- Gastrointestinal upset, including nausea, vomiting, diarrhea or abdominal cramps.
- Headache.
- Dizziness.
- Irritability.
- Some people experience dry skin and a darkening in colour of the skin.
- Plaquenil can be toxic to the retina of the eyes.

Immune system modulators and suppressants

These drugs can alter the number or function of your immune cells. Suppressing the immune system can be very effective for reducing the pain, inflammation and tissue destruction of autoimmune disease, but it may raise the risk of infections and cancer.

The most commonly used drugs in this category include:

- **Cyclophosphamide (Cycloblastin)**

This drug is a type of chemotherapy and is most commonly used for cancers of the immune system, such as lymphoma, myeloma and leukaemia. However, it is also used in autoimmune disease and it's an anti-rejection drug used in organ transplant recipients.

Cyclophosphamide is quite effective in treating lupus related kidney disease. Unfortunately, the side effects can be severe and include nausea, vomiting, infertility and hair loss.

- Mycophenolate mofetil (APO-Mycophenolate, CellCept, Ceptolate, Imulate)

This is a newer drug than cyclophosphamide, with fewer side effects. It is predominantly used for lupus.

- Azathioprine (Imuran)

This is an immunosuppressant that is used in organ transplant recipients and in some autoimmune diseases, particularly lupus, autoimmune liver disease and rheumatoid arthritis. It increases the risk of infections, tumours and also makes your skin more sensitive to sunlight, increasing your risk of burning. In rare cases it may cause inflammation of the white part of the eyes (scleritis).

Monoclonal antibodies

These drugs work in a similar way to the antibodies made by your own immune system. They have the ability to bind to specific immune cells and cause their destruction and clearance from your body. If you can clear some of the immune cells that produce antibodies or inflammatory chemicals, this will reduce the levels of inflammation in your body and reduce tissue destruction.

Examples of monoclonal antibodies are belimumab (Benlysta) and rituximab (Mabthera). These drugs are predominantly used for lupus. They are fairly new drugs, therefore, not all potential side effects are known. They do seem to raise the risk of infections and cancer though.

Methotrexate

Methotrexate was originally used as a chemotherapy drug, but is not often used for cancer these days. Currently, it is mainly used for rheumatoid arthritis, psoriasis, psoriatic arthritis, lupus and other autoimmune diseases. It is generally reserved for use if other therapies have not been successful. Although a low dose is often first line therapy for rheumatoid arthritis.

Methotrexate works by blocking the action of folate in the body. Folate (folic acid) is required for cell division; therefore cells have a reduced capacity to divide in people taking methotrexate. Impairing the ability of specific immune cells to divide can greatly reduce pain, swelling and tissue damage.

Methotrexate is quite toxic to the liver and it can have some serious side effects. Anyone taking this drug needs to have regular liver and kidney function tests, so that any organ damage can be caught early.

Potential side effects of methotrexate include:

- Gastrointestinal upset.
- Increased risk of infections.
- Liver and kidney damage.
- Anaemia.
- Skin problems.

Methotrexate causes folate deficiency, which can have numerous consequences. Most patients benefit from taking a folic acid supplement to counteract this, and it should not reduce the effectiveness of the methotrexate. You'll need to discuss this with your doctor though, so he or she can determine an appropriate dose for you.

If you are taking medication for autoimmune disease, you can still follow the diet and supplement guidelines in this book, as long as you have your own doctor's supervision. You do not need to make a choice of going with orthodox medicine or a natural approach. You can do both; they are complementary.

Ideally, our recommendations will make you healthier so you can slowly wean off your medication, and eventually not require it at all

Please do this under your own doctor's supervision. Throughout this book we have given recommendations that are supported by medical research and that have worked for our patients at our clinics. However, your own doctor knows your medical history and will know what is and isn't appropriate for you.

If you require personalised help, we have a number of services that may benefit you. Please feel free to get in touch with one of our naturopaths on 623 334 3232 or contact@liverdoctor.com

Glossary

Adjuvant

A substance that stimulates the immune system. Adjuvants are added to vaccines to stimulate an immune response that is greater than that induced by the dead or inert virus or bacteria alone. Examples of adjuvants include aluminium, mercury and silicone.

Amylase

A digestive enzyme that breaks down starch.

Antibody

A protein produced by immune cells that recognises a specific molecule and binds to it.

Antigen

A component of a molecule that antibodies bind to.

Anti-nutrient

A substance that prevents the absorption or utilisation of nutrients. Anti-nutrients are predominantly found in grains, legumes, seeds and nuts.

Autoantibody

An antibody that binds to a component of your own body, rather than a foreign harmful substance. Autoantibodies can induce inflammation and tissue damage.

Cortisol

A stress hormone produced by the adrenal glands. Cortisol affects metabolism and weight gain, and it helps to reduce inflammation in the body.

Cytokine

A chemical messenger produced by immune cells. Most cytokines are involved in raising inflammation in the body.

Dysbiosis

Having too much of the wrong microorganisms and not enough of the beneficial microorganisms in the digestive tract.

Enterocyte

The type of cell that lines the gastrointestinal tract.

FODMAPs

Different types of fibers in plant foods that are poorly digested by many people and can cause digestive discomfort in some. Stands for Fermentable Oligosaccharides, Disaccharides, Monosaccharides and Polyols.

Glutathione

A protein made in the body that acts as a powerful antioxidant, detoxifier and anti-inflammatory.

Leaky gut

A situation where the lining of the small intestine becomes more permeable than it should be.

Lectin

A type of protein molecule that has the ability to bind to specific carbohydrates (such as those found on the gastrointestinal lining). Some lectins are capable of causing harm to the digestive and immune system of individuals predisposed to autoimmune disease.

Mitochondria

Tiny organs inside cells that are responsible for producing energy.

Nightshade plants

Plants in the botanical family called solanaceae. Includes potatoes, tomatoes, bell pepper, eggplant, chilli, paprika and goji berries. Substances in these plants can aggravate autoimmune disease in some people.

Prebiotic

Non digestible food (such as dietary fiber) that acts as food for gut microbes.

Probiotic

Beneficial microorganisms that live in your body. Most of them are found in your digestive tract.

Regulatory T cell

A type of immune cell that suppresses the activity of inflammatory cells. It helps to calm down an over active immune system.

Small Intestinal Bacterial Overgrowth (SIBO)

A situation where there is too much bacteria or yeast in the small intestine.

References

1. Australasian Society of Clinical Immunology and Allergy.

2. Progress in Autoimmune Disease Research. The Autoimmune Disease Coordinating Committee Report to Congress. US Dept Health and Human Services, NIH, National Institute of Allergy and Infectious Diseases. Bethesda (MD) 2005

3. Fairweather D, Rose NR. Women and autoimmune disease. Emerg Infect Dis 2004;10:2005-2011

4. Walsh SJ, Rau LM. Autoimmune diseases: a leading cause of death among young and middle aged women in the United States. Am J Public Health 1000 Sep;90(9):1463-6

5. Professor Yehuda Shoenfeld, The Gluten Summit, 2013

6. Willett WC. Balancing lifestyle and genomics research for disease prevention. Science 296(2002):695-98

7. Deeks, S. G., Walker, B. D. Human Immunodeficiency Virus Controllers: Mechanisms of Durable Virus Control in the Absence of Antiretroviral Therapy. Immunity, 2007, 27: 406-416

8. Moon UY, et al. Arthritis Res Ther. 2004;6:R295-302

9. Antonio Gasbarrini, et al. Disappearance of APS after helicobacter pylori eradication. The American Journal of Medicine 2001, 111:163

10. Antibiotics Recommended When Indicated for Treatment of Gulf War Illness/CFIDS/FMS" Prof. Garth L. Nicolson: Intern. J. Medicine 1998; 1: 123-128.

11. Yehuda Shoenfeld 2013

12. Gardner, RM, JF Nyland, IA Silva, AM Ventura, JM deSouza and EK Silbergeld. 2010. Mercury exposure, serum antinuclear/antinucleolar antibodies, and serum cytokine levels in mining populations in

Amazonian Brazil: A cross-sectional study. Environmental Research http://dx.doi.org/10.1016/j.envres.2010.02.001

13. Bigazzi PE, Autoimmunity and heavy metals. Lupus 1994 Dec;3(6):449-53

14. Shoaib BO et al. Human adjuvant disease: presentation as a multiple sclerosis-like syndrome. South Med J 1996;89:179-88

15. Kelly KM et al. Induction of autoimmunity by adjuvant hydrocarbons. Shoenfeld Y, Rose NR, editors. In infection and autoimmunity. 1st edition. San Diego: Elsevier Amsterdam; 2004

16. Lupus. 2012 Feb;21(2):223-30. doi: 10.1177/0961203311430221

17. Ropper A.H., Victor M. 1998. Influenza vaccination and the Guillain–Barre syndrome. New Engl. J. Med. 339: 1845–1846

18. Outi Vaarala. National Institute for Health and Welfare. Department of Vaccinations and Immune Protection, Helsinki, Finland.

19. JAMA. 1997 Oct 8;278(14):1176-8.

20. Miguel A Hernan, et al. Neurology 2004;63:838-842

21. Hepat Mon. Aug 1, 2011; 11(8): 597–598

22. Haugarvoll E et al. Vaccine. 2010; 28:4961-9

23. Datis Kharrazian The Potential Roles of Bisphenol A Pathogenesis in Autoimmunity Autoimmune Diseases Volume 2014 (2014), Article ID 743616

24. Pregnancy hormone could offer simple treatment for MS. New Scientist 2nd May, 2014

25. Alessio Fasano, Leaky gut and autoimmune diseases. Clinical Review of Allergy Immunology 42, February 2012, 71-78

26. Hawrelak, 2013

27. Mark Pimentel MD A New IBS Solution

28. Lombardo et al, 2010

29. Di Stefano M, Miceli E, Missanelli A, Mazzocchi S, Corazza GR. 2005. Absorbable vs. non-absorbable antibiotics in the treatment of small intestine bacterial overgrowth in patients with blind-loop syndrome. Alimentary Pharmacology & Therapeutics, 21:8;985-92. doi: 10.1111/j.1365-2036.2005.02397Di

30. Victor Chedid, et al. Glob Adv Health Med 2014 May;3(3):16-24

31. Ogbolu DO, et al. In vitro antimicrobial properties of coconut oil on Candida species in Ibadan, Nigeria J Med Food. 2007 Jun;10(2):384-7

32. Byron W. Petschow, et al. Susceptibility of Helicobacter pylori to Bactericidal Properties of Medium-Chain Monoglycerides and Free Fatty Acids Antimicrobial Agents and Chemotherapy Feb. 1996, p. 302-306

33. Surawicz, C.M., et al., Treatment of recurrent Clostridium difficile colitis with vancomycin and Saccharomyces boulardii. Am J Gastroenterol, 1989. 84(10): p. 1285-7.

34. Surawicz, C.M., et al., Prevention of antibiotic-associated diarrhea by Saccharomyces boulardii: a prospective study. Gastroenterology, 1989. 96(4): p. 981-8.

35. Buts, J.-P., et al., Stimulation of secretory IgA and secretory component of immunoglobulins in small intestine of rats treated with Saccharomyces boulardii. Dig Dis Sci. 1990 Feb;35(2):251-6

36. Bengmark S. Gut microbiota, immune development and function. Pharmacological Research 2013;69:87-113.

37. Jonathan W. Olson*, Robert J. Maier† Molecular hydrogen as an energy source for Helicobacter pylori Science 29 November 2002: Vol. 298 no. 5599 pp. 1788-1790 DOI: 10.1126/science.1077123

38. Drago S. et al, Gliadin, zonulin and gut permeability: Effects on celiac and non-celiac intestinal mucosa and intestinal cell lines Scand J Gastroenterol. 2006 Apr;41(4):408-19

39. Batchelor AJ, et al. Reduced plasma half-life of radio-labelled 25-hydroxyvitamin D3 in subjects receiving a high-fiber diet. Br J Nutr. 1983 Mar;49(2):213-6.

40. David L J Freed Do dietary lectins cause disease? The evidence is suggestive - and raises possibilities for treatment BMJ. Apr 17, 1999; 318 (7190): 1023-1024.

41. Monetini L, et al. Antibodies to bovine beta-casein in diabetes and other autoimmune diseases. Horm Metab Res. 2002 Aug;34(8):455-9

42. Susan Leech Molecular mimicry in autoimmune disease. Arch Dis Child 1998;79:448-451 doi:10.1136/adc.79.5.448

43. Niebuhr DW, et al. Association between bovine casein antibody and new onset schizophrenia among US military personnel. Schizophr Res. 2011 May;128(1-3):51-5

44. National Digestive Diseases Clearinghouse, National Institutes of Health. NIH Publication no. 09-2751. 2009. http://digestive.niddk.nih. gov/ddiseases/pubs/lactoseintolerance/

45. Aliment Pharmacol Ther. 2005 Nov 1;22(9):789-94.

46. Inflamm Bowel Dis. 2002 Sep;8(5):340-6

47. Ferland G. Vitamin K and the nervous system: an overview of its actions. Adv Nutr 3 (2012):204-12

48. Guerrero-Beltran CE, et al. Protective effect of sulforaphane against oxidative stress: recent advances. Exp Toxicol Pathol 64 (2012):503-508

49. Patty W Siri-Tarino, Meta-analysis of prospective cohort studies evaluating the association of saturated fat with cardiovascular disease Am J Clin Nutr January 13, 2010

50. Nagao K1, Yanagita T. Medium-chain fatty acids: functional lipids for the prevention and treatment of the metabolic syndrome. Pharmacol Res. 2010 Mar;61(3):208-12

51. van der Mei IA, Ponsonby AL, Blizzard L, et al. Regional variation

in multiple sclerosis prevalence in Australia and its association with ambient ultraviolet radiation. Neuroepidemiology 2001; 20:168-174

52. van der Mei IA, Ponsonby AL, Dwyer T, et al. Past exposure to sun, skin phenotype, and risk of multiple sclerosis: case-control study. Bmj 2003; 327:316

53. Freedman DM, et al. Mortality from multiple sclerosis and exposure to residential and occupational solar radiation: a case-control study based on death certificates. Occup Environ Med. 2000 Jun;57(6):418-21

54. Neurology 2011; 76:540-548

55. Cha Kyung, et al. Silibinin Inhibits LPS-Induced Macrophage Activation by Blocking p38 MAPK in RAW 264.7 Cells Biomol Ther (Seoul). Jul 30, 2013; 21(4): 258–263.

56. Dehmlow C et al Hepatology 1996; 23: 749-54

57. Julie S. Jurenka, MT(ASCP) Anti-inflammatory properties of curcumin, a major constituent of Curcuma longa: A review of preclinical and clinical research Alternative Medicine Review volume 14, number 2, 2009

58. Shoskes D, et al. Beneficial effects of the bioflavonoids curcumin and quercetin on early function in cadaveric renal transplantation: a randomized placebo controlled trial. Transplantation 2005;80;1556-1559

59. Roland Gartner, et al. Selenium Supplementation in Patients with Autoimmune Thyroiditis Decreases Thyroid Peroxidase Antibodies Concentrations. The Journal of Clinical Endocrinology and Metabolism Volume 87 Issue 4 - April 1, 2002

60. Turker O, et al. Selenium treatment in autoimmune thyroiditis: 9-month follow-up with variable doses. J Endocrinol. 2006 Jul;190(1):151-6.

61. Tewthanom K et al. Correlation of lipid peroxidation and

glutathione levels with severity of systemic lupus erythematosus: a pilot study from single center. J Pharm Pharm Sci. 2008;11(3):30-4

62. J Lab Clin Med 2002;139:311-5

63. Scott, ME, et al. Zinc deficiency impairs immune responses against parasitic nematode infections at intestinal and systemic sites. Journal of Nutrition 2000; 130(5 Suppl): 1412S-20S.

64. Miller AL. Therapeutic considerations of L-glutamine: a review of the literature. Altern Med Rev 1999;4(4):239-248.

65. Humphreys C. Intestinal permeability assessment. In: Pizzorno JE, Murray MT (eds.). Textbook of natural medicine, 3rd ed (pp 241-9). St Louis, Missouri: Churchill Livingstone Elsevier, 2006

66. Monograph L-glutamine. Altern Med Rev 2001;6(4):406-410

67. Hashimoto M et al. Planta Med 1985;51: 401

68. Vuddanda PR, Chakraborty S, Singh S. Berberine: a potential phytochemical with multispectrum therapeutic activities. Expert Opin Investig Drugs. (2010)

69. Cernáková M, Kostálová D. Antimicrobial activity of berberine--a constituent of Mahonia aquifolium. Folia Microbiol (Praha). (2002)

70. Kaneda Y, et al. In vitro effects of berberine sulphate on the growth and structure of Entamoeba histolytica, Giardia lamblia and Trichomonas vaginalis. Ann Trop Med Parasitol. (1991)

71. Ghosh AK, Bhattacharyya FK, Ghosh DK. Leishmania donovani: amastigote inhibition and mode of action of berberine. Exp Parasitol. (1985)

72. Gu L, et al. Berberine ameliorates intestinal epithelial tight-junction damage and down-regulates myosin light chain kinase pathways in a mouse model of endotoxinemia. J Infect Dis. 2011 Jun 1;203(11):1602-12

73. J Am Coll Nutr. 2002 Dec;21(6):495-505.

74. Michael Ash DO, ND, BSc DipION MIoD The Autoimmune Summit, 2014

75. Mangin M1, Sinha R, Fincher K. Inflammation and vitamin D: the infection connection. Inflamm Res. 2014 Oct;63(10):803-19

76. Leung WC, Hessel S, Méplan C, Flint J, Oberhauser V, Tourniaire F, Hesketh JE, von Lintig J, Lietz G.. Two common single nucleotide polymorphisms in the gene encoding beta-carotene 15,15'-monoxygenase alter beta-carotene metabolism in female volunteers.. FASEB J. 2009 . Apr;23(4):1041-53

Index

A

adjuvant 26, 41, 49, 50, 51, 129, 235, 239

adrenal glands 56, 57, 61, 87, 200, 201, 202, 203, 209, 210, 229, 235

allergies 26, 34, 50, 70, 76, 91, 101, 107, 116, 195

aluminium 40, 41, 49, 149, 235

anti-nuclear antibodies 213

apple cider vinegar 109, 156, 159

auto-antibodies 38, 53, 69, 213

B

berberine 84, 98, 102, 184, 185, 195, 243

betaine HCL 109

bile 67, 81, 84, 91, 105, 106, 110, 111, 113, 160

blood tests 15, 101, 172, 181, 206, 213, 218

bone broth 68, 84, 113, 153, 155, 158, 159, 195, 204

breath test 36, 95, 96, 98

bupleurum 115, 184

C

calcium 86, 141, 158

Candida 76, 81, 83, 88, 101, 102, 153, 160, 240

cholesterol 11, 24, 25, 56, 58, 59, 60, 130, 174, 184, 229

coconut oil 66, 98, 102, 109, 145, 155, 157, 160, 161, 162, 163, 166, 204, 224, 240

celiac disease 17, 19, 29, 30, 31, 34, 53, 63, 64, 69, 75, 78, 79, 90, 94, 109, 111, 112, 117, 119, 120, 122, 126, 128, 168, 174, 176, 197, 209, 213

cortisol 56, 57, 58, 59, 61, 201, 203, 209, 210, 235

cravings 57, 91, 101, 145, 198, 199, 200, 202, 229

C-reactive protein 115, 207

curcumin 177, 242

cytokine 11, 13, 38, 56, 114, 133, 175, 176, 177, 185, 187, 236, 238

D

dairy products 67, 68, 83, 102, 126, 127, 128, 165, 219

die off 98, 103

digestion 66, 69, 81, 86, 88, 89, 104, 105, 108, 109, 111, 112, 125, 131, 138, 149, 158, 160, 195, 198, 212, 226

digestive enzymes 81, 84, 91, 94, 105, 106, 109, 110, 111, 112, 113, 122, 125, 131, 218, 235

E

dysbiosis 81, 82, 83, 84, 88, 104, 105, 112, 119, 198, 207, 213, 236

eggs 34, 66, 83, 130, 131, 165, 166, 188

endotoxin 39, 76, 82, 104, 105, 114, 176, 185, 218, 243

Epstein-Barr virus 31, 35

Erythrocyte Sedimentation Rate (ESR) 191, 206

F

fats 24, 42, 59, 66, 68, 111, 113, 132, 141, 142, 144, 145, 146, 147, 148, 149, 155, 160, 161, 166, 187, 188, 200, 203, 224

fermented foods 85, 93, 113, 149, 150, 152

flare 32, 56, 59, 61, 69, 77, 168, 175, 181, 203, 204, 219, 225

FODMAPs 94, 96, 108, 116, 125, 132, 150, 159, 167, 168, 169

food intolerance 26, 57, 70, 72, 93, 108

food sensitivity 70, 71, 72

fructose 94, 96, 99, 138, 168, 169

G

genes 9, 28, 29, 30, 31, 44, 117, 134

genetic 9, 29, 31, 35, 40, 50, 53, 73, 117, 125

gliadin 118, 122

glutamine 84, 153, 158, 182

gluten 7, 30, 31, 34, 67, 78, 81, 83, 90, 102, 117, 118, 119, 120, 122, 128, 133, 164, 171

glycine 153, 154, 158

grains 67, 68, 69, 81, 83, 102, 117, 118, 119, 120, 121, 129, 135, 142, 164

Guillain Barre syndrome 20, 35, 37, 52

H

Hashimoto's 13, 17, 20, 27, 63, 64, 69

Helicobacter pylori 32, 36, 102, 107, 108, 123, 125, 160

histamine 123, 195, 196, 197, 198

hormones 14, 54, 56, 58, 60, 61, 62, 63, 64, 69, 87, 128, 146

Human Leukocyte Antigen (HLA) 29

I

IgA 182, 183, 195, 213, 240

infection 10, 26, 28, 30, 32, 34, 35, 36, 37, 38, 39, 40, 42, 49, 57, 65, 71, 81, 83, 85, 86, 93, 97, 100, 101, 102, 103, 107, 108, 115, 123, 125, 131, 160

inflammation 8, 13, 14, 25, 34, 37, 38, 40, 43, 58, 61, 62, 66, 70, 77, 84, 86, 88, 89, 90, 100, 104, 105, 110, 112, 114, 120, 124, 126, 128, 133, 136, 138, 143, 144, 146, 149, 163

intestines 30, 34, 67, 68, 70, 73, 74, 77, 79, 82, 86, 88, 90, 91, 92, 94, 95, 96, 97, 99, 108, 116, 118, 119, 120, 124, 128, 133, 136

J

juice 109, 157, 163, 164, 165, 166

L

leaky gut 28, 30, 35, 57, 67, 70, 73, 74, 76, 77, 78, 79, 80, 81, 82, 83, 84, 88, 89, 97, 100, 103, 106, 113, 114, 116, 117, 119, 127, 129, 131, 133, 136, 149, 154, 158, 168

lectins 81, 118, 119, 121, 122, 123, 124, 125

legumes 67, 68, 81, 83, 125, 129, 132, 135, 149, 165, 166

liver 7, 31, 35, 39, 67, 73, 76, 79, 82, 85, 86, 87, 89, 90, 97, 100, 102, 103, 104, 110, 111, 113, 114, 115, 116, 121, 135, 136, 153, 154, 157, 160

lupus 8, 12, 13, 15, 17, 19, 23, 25, 27, 30, 31, 35, 38, 39, 41, 44, 50, 55, 63, 64, 136

M

macrophage 114, 183, 189, 242

magnesium 67, 79, 86, 90, 103, 141, 185

marrow 153, 154, 155, 158, 228

mercury 40, 41, 42, 49, 141, 235, 238

microbiome 85, 86, 87

milk thistle 176

molecular mimicry 32, 38, 49, 81, 126, 131, 241

multiple sclerosis 8, 10, 17, 18, 21, 31, 35, 37, 39, 44, 53, 61, 136, 175

N

naltrexone 190, 191

neutrophil 179, 189, 206

nightshade 72, 83, 129, 130, 138, 165

nutrient 28, 32, 34, 35, 39, 61, 65, 66, 67, 68, 69, 70, 73, 74, 75, 76, 77, 82, 83, 84, 86, 88, 90, 99, 106, 109, 111, 114, 115, 116, 117, 118, 125, 128, 135, 141, 146, 150, 153, 154, 158, 159, 168

O

offal 68, 153, 154

omega 3 fatty acids 187

P

parasites 32, 76, 81, 109, 182, 192, 193, 194

PCR test 40, 194

prebiotic 87, 135, 170, 237

probiotic 34, 85, 87, 93, 149, 150, 152

progesterone 18, 57, 58, 59, 60, 61, 62

R

recipes 151, 152, 157, 170, 171

red meat 141, 142, 143, 165

S

Saccharomyces boulardii 102, 195, 240

saponins 81, 125, 129

selenium 37, 42, 69, 115, 141, 178, 179, 181, 215, 216, 222, 224, 226, 242

SIBO (Small Intestinal Bacterial Overgrowth) 83-84, 91-99, 107, 127, 185, 197, 218, 220

silicone 43, 44, 45, 46, 47, 48, 49, 54, 235

sleep 12, 14, 25, 26, 39, 40, 79, 103, 104, 115, 131, 154, 158, 184, 185, 186, 193, 196, 199, 201, 202, 203, 204, 205, 216, 217, 218, 223, 224, 225

soy 66, 122, 125, 165, 188, 196, 215

steroid 58, 59, 60, 61, 101, 173, 174, 184, 203, 219, 228, 229, 230

St Mary's thistle 115, 176

stomach acid 67, 81, 84, 91, 93, 94, 105, 106, 107, 108, 109, 112, 123, 131, 158, 195, 197, 212

stress 9, 12, 14, 25, 28, 32, 35, 38, 55, 56, 57, 58, 61, 81, 82, 86, 100, 103, 108, 112, 115, 134, 136, 170, 172, 180, 181, 186, 190, 201, 202, 203, 204, 209, 214, 215, 216, 225, 235, 241

T

thyroid 8, 11, 13, 17, 31, 41, 54, 62, 63, 64, 69, 82, 87, 122, 125

V

vaccination 41, 49, 50, 51, 52, 53, 54, 239

vitamin A 81, 84, 136, 141, 188, 189, 195, 226

vitamin C 37, 136, 181, 183, 189, 190, 202

vitamin D 37, 69, 79, 90, 111, 121, 141, 142, 173, 174, 175, 186, 189, 210, 215, 216, 218, 220, 222, 223, 226, 241, 244

W

wheat 108, 119, 120, 121, 122, 123, 164

Z

zonulin 77, 78, 119, 120, 240

From the desk of Dr Cabot

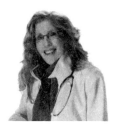

Liver Formulas

There are hundreds of liver formulas and tonics sold all over the world and indeed they have been used with great benefit in China and Europe for thousands of years.

I wanted patients to be able to take everything they needed in one formula thus avoiding the expense and uncertainty of having to swallow multiple individual supplements.

This inspired me to develop the LivaTone range of liver tonics, which had multiple essential herbs and antioxidant nutrients in the correct amounts all combined together in one capsule or powder. The LivaTone formulas became a registered trademark so patients could know that they were getting my original formula with proven and safe ingredients.

Subsequently, several liver tonics appeared on the market with similar names such as Liver Tone or Livertone etc., but they are very different formulas to the original LivaTone formulas and they do not have my name on them.

For more information see www.liverdoctor.com or phone our friendly and professional naturopaths in Phoenix Arizona on 1 623 334 3232.

LivaTone Plus

LivaTone Plus is a powerful liver tonic that combines the pure extract of the herb milk thistle (St Mary's Thistle) with -

- All the B group vitamins including activated folic acid (folinic acid) and methyl-cobalamin (B 12); these are essential for healthy liver function and detoxification

- The most important liver amino acids glutamine, glycine, glutathione, NAC and taurine, which are needed for efficient liver detoxification and liver protection

- An effective dose of the important antioxidant vitamins namely vitamins C, E and natural beta-carotene

- The minerals selenium and zinc; these promote detoxification in the liver and reduce liver inflammation.

LivaTone Plus is a powerful synergistic formula that has been designed to support the detoxification pathways within the liver. Specific nutrients and herbs can stimulate the repair and renewal of damaged liver cells. They also enhance the liver's ability to break down toxic chemicals via the Step One and Step Two detoxification processes.

Ingredients in LivaTone Plus

Glutamine

This amino acid is high in organic sulfur and is required for the Step Two liver detoxification pathway which breaks down and eliminates drugs and toxic chemicals. Glutamine is converted in the body into glutamic acid, which along with the amino acids cysteine and glycine, is converted into glutathione. Glutathione is an extremely powerful liver protector.

N-Acetyl-Cysteine

This amino acid is a proven liver protector with a long history of clinical trials and is the main precursor of glutathione.

Taurine

This amino acid is essential for the production of bile. The liver uses taurine to eliminate toxins and drugs from the body through the bile. Taurine helps the liver to excrete excessive cholesterol out of the body through the bile and thus is an aid for weight control. Taurine is called the detoxifying amino acid and is continually required by the liver.

Glycine

This amino acid is required for the synthesis of bile salts and is used by the liver to detoxify chemicals in the Step Two detoxification pathways.

Antioxidants

LivaTone Plus contains the most important liver antioxidants NAC, vitamin E, vitamin C, carotenoids, selenium and zinc.

LivaTone Plus also contains green tea extract which has antioxidant properties.

Antioxidants prevent free radicals from oxidizing the cell membranes in the liver, which prevents cell damage. During the liver detoxification of toxins and drugs, large amounts of free radicals are generated in the liver; antioxidants are needed to prevent these from causing liver damage. Vitamin E has been proven to reduce scarring in the liver, which can lead to cirrhosis.

B Group Vitamins

LivaTone Plus contains all the B group vitamins – namely vitamins B1, B2, B3, B5, B6, B12, Folinic Acid, Biotin and Inositol. These vitamins are essential for the production of energy in the liver and many people with liver problems feel excessively tired. The liver is the metabolic factory of the body and thus optimal function is vital for you to feel continually energized. Many people who consume excess alcohol or suffer high stress are deficient in B vitamins; this increases their risk of liver damage.

Vitamin B12 (in the form of methylcobalamin) and activated folic acid (folinic acid) are required for the liver to perform methylation, which inactivates excess estrogens and toxins, which can otherwise build up and cause cancer. Interestingly, many strict vegans are deficient in Vitamin B12 and the amino acid taurine; this can result in liver dysfunction.

LivaTone Plus contains broccoli powder. Broccoli is a cruciferous vegetable, which contains liver healing substances (such as indoles, thiols and sulfur compounds).

Milk Thistle (also known as St Mary's Thistle)

The clinically effective dose of the herb Milk Thistle has been proven to reduce liver damage in many European clinical trials. The active component of milk thistle is called silymarin and 420mg of pure silymarin is required daily to get good results during the initial stages of taking a liver formula. The length of time you need to take this dose for depends upon the state of your liver.

Milk thistle has been used for more than 2000 years to treat liver diseases and is a safe nontoxic herb. Milk Thistle does not cause any side effects and its young fresh leaves were once eaten as a food in Europe.

The silymarin in Milk Thistle protects the membranes of the liver cells and stimulates the production of new healthy liver cells to replace damaged liver cells. Silymarin can improve protein synthesis in the liver and helps the liver filter to remove dangerous toxins.

Research shows that silymarin from Milk Thistle protects against glutathione depletion and increases liver glutathione, thus supporting liver detoxification and protection from free radicals. Milk Thistle stimulates the production of bile, which is important since bile acts as a way to excrete toxins into the intestines. This has been demonstrated in a pilot study when Milk Thistle, combined with vitamin E reduced signs of fatty liver.

Modern pharmacological technology has enabled all these ingredients to be combined together in powder or capsules; this makes it much easier to take and much more affordable.

This combination of high dose pure silymarin and all the required vitamins and minerals and amino acids, is called LivaTone Plus. Begin with one capsule twice daily or one teaspoon daily for 2 weeks. Thereafter increase the dose to two capsules twice daily or one teaspoon of the powder twice daily. Maintenance doses vary from 2 to 4 capsules daily. It is best taken with food.

The powder can be stirred into fresh juices or water and although the B vitamins give it a characteristic smell, it is not unpleasant to take. The capsules are best taken with food, but if you forget, it is acceptable to take them on an empty stomach.

Choosing a liver formula

When you have a compromised liver it is vital to take a formula that contains an effective dosage of the active proven ingredients. The ingredients should be standardized and pure so you know that you are getting the correct dosage.

So when choosing your liver formula, choose wisely and check the types and the amounts of the ingredients in the different formulations available - you may get a surprise! Some liver formulas contain a large selection of herbs but they are only small amounts and they do not have any antioxidant vitamins, minerals or amino acids at all.

It's also good to get professional advice when choosing a liver formula. For more information call our Health Advisory Service on 1 623 334 3232.

It is also important to know that the liver tonic you decide to take is –

- Made in a laboratory that has obtained Good Manufacturing Procedures (GMP) certification and FDA approval

- Made in a laboratory that is audited by an independent not for profit body such as The National Science Foundation - see http://www.nsf.gov/

- Analyzed by a laboratory to validate the identity, purity and amounts of its contained ingredients

- Under stability studies to test that its active ingredients last as long as their stated shelf life (expiry date) on the container

- Free of artificial binders and fillers

- Vegetarian so that the gelatin capsule cannot transmit bovine diseases

LivaTone Plus satisfies all these criteria.

Note: Some other forms of liver products on the market contain silymarin mixed with lecithin. This is most commonly diluted with phosphatidylcholine which comes from lecithin. This is usually two thirds phosphatidylcholine and only one third silybin. This would provide only 80mg of silybin per capsule. This is often promoted as being superior to products which contain pure silymarin and I do not agree with this.

LivaTone Plus has been tested in a clinical study of patients with fatty liver and was found to be safe and effective. More information on this study is available at www.liverdoctor.com and click "Fatty liver study".

Liver formulas are helpful if you –

- Have a chronic viral infection of the liver

- Are using prescription drugs – these must be broken down by the liver and many people are taking several drugs every day, which greatly increases the workload of the liver

- Are using over the counter drugs, especially pain killers or acetaminophen (paracetamol) - these must be broken down by the liver and can be particularly liver toxic, if excessive or daily doses are used.

The combination of acetaminophen with coffee is especially toxic for the liver in those with hepatitis B or C.

- Drink ten or more glasses of alcohol a week - over 18 million Americans abuse alcohol, making it one of the most common causes of liver disease in America.

- Smoke cigarettes

- Consume sugar, fast foods, chemical food additives and/or microwaved cooked foods

- Live in a major city – where you are exposed to automobile exhausts, factory smog, crowded dirty places, water chlorination, fluoride and heavy metals etc.

- Are over 45 years of age - as you get older the various tubes and ducts leading from and to your liver, as well as the internal liver filter itself, often become dirty and/or clogged. They become laden with unhealthy fats, toxins, gallstones, sludge, hardened tissues and waste products of metabolism

- Drink soda pops and/or diet sodas containing artificial sweeteners, especially the sweetener aspartame – see www. dorway.com

- Are exposed to toxic chemicals and pollutants such as - insecticides, some antiperspirants, solvents, glues, aerosol sprays, some detergents, ammonia, hair dyes, nail varnish etc.

- Have high cholesterol and/or triglycerides

- Have skin problems

There are many other reasons that would make it wise to take a liver tonic on a regular daily basis or at the very least, twice a year for a two month course each time. This is especially true in the 21st Century when the world has become increasingly polluted and crowded, and liver infections are increasing.

Your liver processes most of the approximately 900 million pounds of toxic chemicals and drugs released into the environment every year. An overload of these toxins can easily wear out your liver and leave you prone to developing a range of health problems.

Be careful with pain killers, especially acetaminophen (paracetamol), which can damage your liver.

It is well known that overdosing on this popular painkiller can cause liver damage and death via liver necrosis and acute liver failure. A study, in the Journal of the American Medical Association, reported the highest recommended dose of Tylenol® (acetaminophen or paracetamol) can quickly increase liver enzymes in healthy adults. Elevated enzymes are the first sign of liver damage. If you drink alcohol or have kidney problems, the risk of liver damage from paracetamol is increased significantly.

Your liver is under attack 24 hours, 7 days a week, so it's vital to support its functions and reduce its risk of damage. If you have a clean and unclogged liver, you will have extra years of energetic living to enjoy.

Sandra Cabot MD

Do you suffer with stubborn health problems?

Sandra Cabot MD has written over 30 health books covering many of the health problems facing people all over the world today.

Her award winning Liver Cleansing Diet book has helped many thousands of people regain their health and helped them to better understand the vital role that liver health plays in their daily lives. This popular book has sold over 2 million copies and been translated into six languages and continues to be one of her best selling books.

Dr Cabot's books provide holistic solutions for:

- Menopause
- Weight excess
- Hormonal imbalances
- Chronic fatigue
- Adrenal exhaustion
- Thyroid problems
- Rapid aging
- Mood disorders and stress
- Endometriosis
- Headaches
- Fibromyalgia
- Painful sexual intercourse

I have been practicing medicine for almost 40 years and, during that time, have seen patients heal themselves from so called "incurable" diseases as well as dozens of common and chronic health problems.

The truth is, in most cases, serious illnesses do not happen overnight. Your body produces warning signs and symptoms of a potential or evolving health problem.

I hope you enjoy reading my books and, by better understanding your personal health problems, you are able to be more proactive in helping your body to heal.

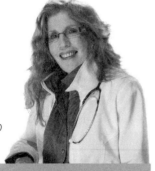

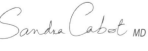 MD

Full list of titles available:

- Alzheimer's - Protect your brain
- Bird Flu - A survival guide
- Body Shaping Diet
- Boost Your Energy
- Breast Cancer Prevention Guide
- Cholesterol: The real truth
- Diabetes Type 2: You can reverse it naturally
- Endometrosis - Your best chance to cure it *(only available as eBook)*
- Fatty Liver - You can reverse it
- Gluten - Is it making you sick or fat?
- Healhy Bowel Healthy Body
- Help for Depression and Anxiety
- Hepatitis and AIDS - How to fight them naturally *(only available as eBook)*
- Hormone Replacement - The real truth
- Hormones - Don't let them ruin your life
- How Not to Kill Your Husband
- How to Increase Your Sex Drive Naturally
- Infertility: The hidden causes
- Liver Cleansing Diet - revised 2014
- Magnesium - The miracle mineral
- Raw Juices Can Save Your Life
- Save Your Gallbladder - and what to do if you have already lost it
- Tired of Not Sleeping?
- Want to Lose Weight but Hooked on Food?
- Your Thyroid Problems Solved

Many of the above books are also available as eBooks